Relieving Pelvic Pain
During and After Pregnancy

Written by a physical therapist who has experienced pregnancy-related pelvic pain firsthand, *Relieving Pelvic Pain During and After Pregnancy* provides a practical blend of traditional and novel treatment approaches that will help women regain control over their bodies and their lives. Cecile Röst draws upon personal experience, patient interaction, and her own research to deliver a fresh look at this frequently misunderstood condition in a way that benefits both patients and therapists alike.

— Anne Ahlman, MPT

About the Author

CECILE RÖST is the mother of three children. In 1985 she graduated as a physiotherapist from the Academie voor Fysiotherapie Jan van Essen, in Amsterdam, Netherlands. During her third pregnancy she resolved her own pelvic instability by developing special exercises to treat the condition. Since then she has used this method to treat patients with pelvic pain and pelvic instability. She also presents workshops and lectures to train fitness trainers, nurses, midwives, physiotherapists, and doctors on the use of her method of therapy.

Relieving Pelvic Pain
During and After Pregnancy

How Women Can Heal
Chronic Pelvic Instability

Cecile C. M. Röst

With contributions from

Christine Buttinger   Jacqueline Kaiser   Pieter van de Vaart

Karen Jongenelen   Anne van Ommeren

Hunter House PUBLISHERS

PROJECT CREDITS

Cover Design: Peri Poloni-Gabriel

Book Production: John McKercher

Illustrator: Peter Slominski

Translator: Joan MacDonald

Developmental Editor: Nancy Faass, MPH

Copy Editor: Kelley Blewster

Proofreader: John David Marion

Indexer: Nancy D. Peterson

Acquisitions Editor: Jeanne Brondino

Editor: Alexandra Mummery

Senior Marketing Associate: Reina Santana

Rights Coordinator: Candace Groskreutz

Interns: Amy Hagelin, Alexi Ueltzen,
    Julia Wang

Customer Service Manager:
    Christina Sverdrup

Order Fulfillment: Washul Lakdhon

Administrator: Theresa Nelson

Computer Support: Peter Eichelberger

Publisher: Kiran S. Rana

Ordering

Trade bookstores in the U.S. and Canada please contact
Publishers Group West
1700 Fourth St., Berkeley CA 94710
Phone: (800) 788-3123   Fax: (800) 351-5073

For bulk orders please contact
Special Sales
Hunter House Inc., PO Box 2914, Alameda CA 94501-0914
Phone: (510) 899-5041   Fax: (510) 865-4295
E-mail: sales@hunterhouse.com

Individuals can order our books by calling **(800) 266-5592**
or from our website at **www.hunterhouse.com**

*This book is dedicated
to all who have participated
in the empowering search for relief of pelvic pain.*

*Regaining control of one's body
is a mighty feeling.*

Hunter House Inc., Publishers
PO Box 2914
Alameda CA 94501-0914

LIBRARY OF CONGRESS CATALOGING-IN-PUBLICATION DATA
Röst, Cecile C. M.
[Bekkenpijn tijdens en na de zwangerschap. English]
Relieving pelvic pain during and after pregnancy : how women can heal
chronic pelvic instability /
Cecile C.M. Röst ; with contributions from Christine Buttinger... [et al.]. — 1st ed.
p. cm.
Includes bibliographical references and index.
ISBN-13: 978-0-89793-480-0 (pbk)
ISBN-13: 978-0-89793-547-0 (ebook)
1. Pelvic pain—Treatment. 2. Pregnancy. I. Buttinger, Christine. II. Title.
RG483.P44R67 2006
618.2—dc22   2006020901

Manufactured in the United States of America

9 8 7 6 5 4 3 2   First Edition   13 14 15 16 17

Contents

Part II: Relieving Pelvic Pain Through Exercise

Part III: Daily Activities

Part IV: Pregnancy and Beyond

Part V: Scientific Research and Clinical Information for Therapists

Foreword

Pelvic instability in pregnant women seems to be responsible for an escalating increase in pain complaints reported in the lower body and legs. These are complaints that only a few decades ago were scarce or at least not often reported to health-care providers. Still, the complaints are real. These women are in pain. However, research has not yet discovered the actual cause of their pain. What's known is that an interaction between hormones, changes in the pelvic joints, and a woman's state of mind contribute to the syndrome. Until we know exactly what the actual cause of pelvic pain is, health-care workers must try to help pregnant women, women during childbirth, and new mothers who are in pain. As midwives, doctors, and gynecologists, we can do this by approaching the subject of pelvic instability in a serious way. We can refer women with pelvic pain or dysfunction to a physiotherapist who specializes in treatment of this condition. A unified treatment approach does not yet exist; therefore, it is important that the physiotherapist take the complaint seriously and specialize in its treatment.

Cecile Röst is a physiotherapist, an orthopedic-manual therapist, and the mother of three children. She experienced pelvic instability during her own pregnancies. As a health-care professional, she knows just how painful the condition can be and how little help women may get for it. Using her own experience and insight, she first tested the method outlined in this book on herself. In this way she gained the knowledge required to deal with pelvic instability and to reduce the pain and disability it can cause. I have seen pregnant women and new mothers benefit from Cecile's treatment protocol. This book is a welcome addition to what's currently being offered, even though we have a long way to go before we have clear insight into the root cause of pregnancy-related pelvic pain or instability.

Until that time we *must* help women with pelvic pain!

— Bart van der Lugt
Gynecologist, Kennemer Hospital (Gasthuis), Haarlem, Netherlands

Acknowledgments

Over the past ten years it has been fantastic to be able to help so many families and to observe women in difficult circumstances bravely carry on, full of trust in the future, fighting for themselves and their families.

I am very grateful for the unflagging support of midwives and doctors. They sent my colleagues and me more than three thousand patients to engage in a "new" therapy. Hundreds of colleagues traveled a long distance to visit my practice or took courses so they could better help their patients. Many thanks go to the University of Rotterdam for its generous support, especially to Prof. Dr. Koes, Dr. Verhagen, and Jacqueline Kaiser, M.S., who helped me with scientific research and publishing. Two large studies, published in *Spine* and in *Acta Obstetricia et Gynecologica Scandinavica,* were the result of five years of data collection (1997–2002).

This book has become what it is thanks to the cooperation and contribution of many patients, scientists, and caregivers. The illustrator and the editors did a great job of making the book a real support for so many women.

My experiences in the past years—in private and in my practice—have taken an enormous toll on the people in my life. Their good wishes, support, and cooperation have been huge. Thanks very much, everyone!

Important Note

The material in this book is intended to provide a review of information regarding pregnancy-related pelvic pain and instability. Every effort has been made to provide accurate and dependable information. The contents of this book have been compiled through clinical research and in consultation with medical professionals. However, health-care professionals have differing opinions, and advances in medical and scientific research are made very quickly, so some of the information may become outdated.

Therefore, the publisher, authors, and editors, as well as the professionals quoted in the book, cannot be held responsible for any error, omission, or dated material. The authors and publisher assume no responsibility for any outcome of applying the information in this book in a program of self-care or under the care of a licensed practitioner. If you have questions concerning the application of the information described in this book, consult a qualified health-care professional.

Introduction

This book was written to help pregnant women and new mothers who are experiencing pelvic pain regain control of their bodies.

Over the course of the last decade, thousands of women have been treated with the exercises described in this book. In addition to my work with patients, I have trained many physiotherapists in the Netherlands and Belgium in this technique.

The effectiveness of these methods has been confirmed in a series of studies that followed the progress of hundreds of women with pelvic pain. More than 90 percent of these patients were able to overcome pelvic pain and its related symptoms.

My own interest in this topic began in 1996 when I suffered from pelvic instability during my third pregnancy (just as I had during the first two pregnancies). From my own experience I know how anxiety-provoking and frustrating it can be when your legs refuse to cooperate and something as ordinary as sitting down or turning over in bed becomes painful. It is especially terrible if this occurs while you're relatively young and beginning a part of your life during which you want to care for your new family and be successful at your job.

In spite of my pain, I continued to work as much as possible in my physiotherapy practice. By practicing yoga I discovered an exercise that seemed to diminish the pain. Trying different exercises and yoga positions, I eventually discovered methods by which I could treat pelvic pain and dysfunction.

I have now taught these exercises to other women for ten years. I have seen firsthand that it is possible to treat pelvic discomfort, even during pregnancy. Since 1996 I have helped more than three thousand women in my practice. In addition, through the work of my colleagues, these exercises have been success-fully taught to thousands of other women in Europe.

Research on This Approach

Two articles have been published in medical journals based on the research de-scribed in Part V of this book (Röst et al. 2004 and 2006). The first study ana-lyzes data on 870 pregnant women with pelvic problems. The second describes a follow-up study with 430 women. These women were treated during their pregnancy with the methods described in this book. They filled out an expanded questionnaire an average of eighteen months after delivery.

In the interim between the two studies, a large number of women from the original study had become pregnant and delivered another child; they were also included in the second study. In this follow-up study, only 10 percent of the 430 women still had symptoms and felt limited in at least one of their daily activities, or experienced new symptoms associated with a subsequent pregnancy. None required the use of a wheelchair or crutches. Of the women in the follow-up study who filled out the questionnaire, 98 percent experienced some benefit from the exercises they did while pregnant.

Anna's Story

Anna is one of the women who came to me for physiotherapy to treat pelvic pain and instability. She sent me the following letter when she was at the end of her pregnancy, waiting for the delivery to start:

> I first had symptoms when I was twenty-five weeks pregnant. The symp-toms began with a heavy, dull pain in my pelvic area when I got up to go to the bathroom in the middle of the night. After a few days I started to have difficulty walking. Within a week, the symptoms were much worse and I could climb the stairs only with great effort.
>
> My midwife referred me to a physiotherapist, who prescribed rest and showed me the best way to turn over in bed while I was resting or sleep-ing. Still, the symptoms became much worse. The physiotherapist told me to take as much rest as I needed and, if necessary, to use crutches. Even-tually I couldn't walk without crutches, and I ended up in a wheelchair. I was disappointed to realize that there would be no more enjoyable shop-ping trips or bike rides for the duration of my pregnancy.

One day, while I was wheeling around the city, another pregnant woman asked me if I was in a wheelchair because of pelvic instability problems. She told me that her physiotherapist had helped her with this condition. My boyfriend insisted that I call the physiotherapist, Cecile Röst.

According to Cecile, the problems I was having were the result of poor pelvic posture, and my posture was only being made worse by resting in bed and by using crutches and a wheelchair. After my first treatment with her, I felt much more supple, but I also experienced some pain. For the first two days I didn't feel better—in fact, I felt a little worse—but I faithfully performed the exercises as she had recommended. On the third day I began to feel a bit better, and I could walk small distances without crutches. Within two and a half weeks my worst symptoms were gone.

It's now a month later and everything is going well. People who saw me before are surprised at how well I am doing and how comfortably I can walk. I can climb stairs without a problem. I'm no longer worried about my baby's birth and the future. Altogether, I'm a happy woman.

I got a card from Anna three weeks after her baby's birth, saying, "Everything is going really well. Yesterday I walked almost two miles along the beach. Not bad!"

How to Use This Book

Parts I through IV of the book are for the patient. By reading this material, you can learn what my patients have learned. By faithfully performing the exercises, you can reap the same benefits they've enjoyed. Treating this problem is not just about reducing pain; it's about regaining the ability to use your body efficiently. Once your body is functioning as it should, the pain should diminish and eventually disappear.

The book can also be used by physiotherapists and other health-care practitioners. Part V is specifically addressed to the physiotherapist. It describes my research and analyzes the findings, provides guidelines for the first consultation with a pelvic pain patient, and outlines a treatment protocol.

Typically only a few treatment sessions are required, usually two to four during pregnancy. When women come for therapy after delivery, fifteen treatments are needed, at most. None of the women I have treated still use aids such as pelvic slings or wheelchairs, and they now have little or no pain.

In addition to treating pregnant women and new mothers, this approach has been used by other women who have experienced problems as a result of accident or injury. Colleagues have even told me that they've successfully used the techniques on patients of both sexes with chronic low-back pain or tendonitis of the adductor muscles. The time it takes to completely heal depends on the duration of the complaints and the severity of the disability before beginning therapy.

I asked twenty-five of the women whom I have treated to write something for this book, and all have done so. Excerpts from their letters appear in Parts I through IV. I used the letters as they were written (lightly edited for clarity) but changed the women's names to protect their privacy. The number of treatments each patient underwent is noted.

I have tracked the results of my work and have included my findings in Part V. Everyone I've spoken with was initially skeptical of my program because the exercises are so simple to perform and do not cause that much pain (after the first session the pain diminishes). Now, however, quite a few doctors, therapists, midwives, and pregnancy-exercise instructors are adopting these methods and are quite enthusiastic about this approach. I hope this book will serve to share my knowledge and experience with even more people.

Some patients will be able to use this book without someone else's help. More often, a physiotherapist's help may be necessary to implement these exercises, especially when the patient is experiencing a great deal of pain or anxiety. Do not hesitate to show this book to your health-care professional; the book's purpose is to help as many patients as possible.

Finally, patients who consult this book should heed the following points:

1. If any of the exercises are difficult to perform, it is advisable to perform them under the supervision of a physiotherapist.

2. Consult a doctor for a diagnosis first. The doctor can refer you to a physiotherapist who specializes in the treatment of pelvic dysfunction.

3. Even if a physiotherapist first teaches you how to perform the at-home exercises, for continuing success you will need to be regular and consistent in your exercise program.

4. If you do not improve or if you get worse, you should definitely talk to your doctor or physiotherapist.

PART I

For the Patient:
The Basics about
Pregnancy-Related Pelvic Pain

What Is Pelvic Instability?

How Do You Recognize Pelvic Dysfunction?

What Causes Pregnancy-Related Pelvic Pain? A Closer Look

Anxiety and Pain: A Vicious Cycle

1

What Is Pelvic Instability?

Janet, whose daughter was a year old when she wrote the following account, underwent nine treatments for pelvic pain.

> *On April 10, 1996, my healthy, beautiful daughter, Heather, was born. Before the birth I had experienced some pain in my lower back and pelvis but thought it was a normal part of pregnancy and paid little attention to it. After the birth, I spent the first few months in a happy daze, ignoring all the pain. Then I had to go back to work in August, and the pain became worse. I went to the doctor and he recommended physiotherapy, but the therapy just made the pain even worse. After several treatments I felt that I was regressing. Then I went to a therapist who used chiropractic techniques. He saw right away that it was not my back but my pelvis that was the problem.*
>
> *He suggested a pelvic sling and contacted my doctor about sending me to the hospital. There, after undergoing many X rays, scans, and other tests, I spent four weeks in a cast. It was pure hell because you can't do anything—you can't even sit or lie down comfortably. The cast didn't fit well: When I did lie down, there was enough room between my body and my cast to prop a towel in. With the support gone, the pain became unbearable.*
>
> *After two weeks, a groove was sawed in the cast and I was given a pelvic sling so I could turn over in the evening. After four weeks, nothing that had been done had had any effect at all, and the pain continued.*
>
> *I reached the point where I could only hobble around the house. I could only go outside in a wheelchair. I could not care for my own daughter and*

had to have someone in the house day and night to do everything. My husband not only took care of Heather and me, but he was also there for me emotionally. He cheered me up after all my crying spells.

Finally I went to see Cecile, who had a program for treating pelvic pain. Two days after the first exercise session, I noticed an improvement. I had not seen any improvement for months. In fact, I had only seen things get worse. One week after beginning the exercises, I could already walk better. I didn't need my pelvic sling anymore; nor did I need the wheelchair. Now, after nine treatments (three and a half months later), I can climb stairs again, walk for a while, ride my bike for a while, take care of my daughter, and do some light housework. Sitting up straight for more than a half hour or standing for long isn't quite possible yet, but I am so happy that I have gotten this far.

Yvonne had experienced pelvic pain for several years. When she first saw me for treatment she still walked with crutches. She noticed significant improvement after only four sessions.

It's hard to believe that it could take six years of seeking treatment for pain and dysfunction before finally meeting someone who knows what's going on in your body and can really help you. After all this time, it's great to be pain free!

As you can see from the stories of Janet and Yvonne, pelvic pain can be debilitating and frustrating—even agonizing. What is it, and what causes it?

First, let's deal with terminology. The term "pelvic instability" is nowadays often replaced by the term "pregnancy-related pelvic (or pelvic girdle) pain," which is a much better description of this symptomatic disorder. It has also been called "peripartum pelvic pain"—pelvic pain that occurs around the time of delivery. The term "pelvic instability" is best used once a formal diagnosis of such is made by a physiotherapist or doctor. In Parts I through IV of this book I've used the terms "pelvic pain," "pregnancy-related pelvic pain," and "pelvic instability" somewhat interchangeably. If you're interested in a slightly more clinical discussion of terminology, see Chapter 12.

Pelvic pain involves the bones, joints, nervous system, and muscles of the pelvic and lower-back area. Although the pelvis appears to be a fixed circle of bone, it is actually made up of three separate bones joined together (see Figure 1.1 on the next page):

- ❏ the two hipbones (the ilia)
- ❏ the backbone in the lower spine (the sacrum), wedged between the hipbones

A fourth bone, the tailbone (coccyx), is involved in some cases of pregnancy-related pelvic pain.

There are also three joints:

- ❏ the pubic joint (the pubic symphysis, connecting both hipbones on the front side)
- ❏ two joints in the lower back area on either side of the sacrum, known as the sacroiliac (SI) joints

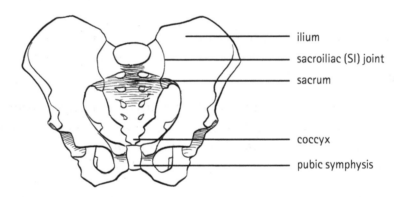

ilium

sacroiliac (SI) joint

sacrum

coccyx

pubic symphysis

1.1. The pelvis

The bones form a ring that is held together with ligaments and cartilage, which relax and stretch in response to hormonal changes during pregnancy in order to expand the birth canal area during delivery. This results in the lengthening and weakening of the ligaments of the pelvic joints, the connective fascia, and the surrounding muscles, which all provide stability to the pelvic ring. As a result, the bones may shift and become misaligned, causing pain and interfering with the ability to move properly. Since the musculoskeletal system is interrelated, this misalignment may ultimately affect the entire body. Functional movements that were once taken for granted, such as moving from sitting to standing, reaching to put things away, or simply getting out of bed in the morning, may all become difficult and painful.

Who Experiences Pregnancy-Related Pelvic Pain?

Having an unstable pelvis is a normal condition in pregnancy and doesn't necessarily lead to pain; in fact, it is a useful condition that facilitates giving birth. The research of Leonie Damen has shown that pregnant women who experience pelvic pain have differing amounts of laxity between their right and left sacroiliac joints as compared to other pregnant women. A large difference in laxity may cause a displacement of the ilium or the portion of the sacrum that has the most freedom to move. Thus, it is thought that pain arises from the misalignment that occurs as a result of a slightly shifted ilium and/or sacrum into a badly recognized position. As a result of the "new" position in the sacroiliac joint, one will unconsciously try to restore the situation, and muscles will tense and pull within or around the pelvis. This will cause pelvic pain if the wrong muscles try to do the correcting. Tension in the pelvic-floor muscles or in the muscles of the inside of the leg (adductor muscles) will worsen the misaligment and provoke pain.

Women who swam a lot during their youth have significantly more complaints than other patients. I think one of the reasons behind this is that these women have developed a motor pattern that involves a strong use of the pelvic-floor and adductor muscles.

Women who experienced low-back pain before pregnancy or who have demanding jobs that require them to stand for much of the day, such as nurses or physical therapists, are at greater risk of experiencing pelvic pain while pregnant and also of having to endure a prolonged recovery. This could be because the muscle system that should be used in forward-bending or lifting activities has not been sufficiently trained. In other words, poor posture can lead not only to low-back pain but also to pelvic pain!

You can compare pregnancy-related pelvic pain with a train derailment. The train is the ilium, which has derailed from the sacrum. The railway system (the body) is paralyzed at once, and the railway workers (nerves and muscles) panic. Transportation (body movement) must continue, so buses are called in (muscles that would normally carry out other functions), sent by the railroad's central administration (the brain). Once the train is put back on track (via symmetry exercises) and the damage is repaired (during the postpregnancy period), the panic subsides. Traffic returns to normal, and slowly the malfunctions (pain complaints) disappear.

The derailment between the sacrum and the ilium causes the muscles and joints to send the wrong signals, which makes a patient incapable of instinctively feeling or sensing how she should move. The loss of contact between the surfaces of the joints results in unnatural movement patterns and forces the muscles into inappropriate positions. The result is that some muscles tense up while others become weakened. This displacement of the pelvis may have already occurred before a woman became pregnant, but it usually takes place during the pregnancy or delivery.

A derailment doesn't just confuse train traffic; it affects the entire system, which can become overwhelmed when certain parts of the body must accommodate jobs normally done by other areas of the body. Other people may have to take over some of the woman's daily functions.

How Pelvic Pain Can Affect Your Life

Having a child always prompts many life changes, and it is even more difficult to make the required adjustments when the new mother is in constant pain and cannot function; she is not able to take care of her child, cannot enjoy physical intimacy, and requires a great deal of help.

Fortunately, most of my patients tell me that their relationships with their partners improve rapidly once they regain control of their bodies. If it doesn't look like a couple is going to be able to overcome this setback, it may be a good idea for them to discuss the problem with a doctor or a marriage counselor.

Take heart. This book will help you to prevent big trouble and regain normal functioning whenever your pelvis slips out of order.

2

How Do You Recognize
Pelvic Dysfunction?

Ellen is another patient for whom it took several years to pinpoint the cause of her problems, which shows how difficult it can be to define these conditions, particularly when they develop over time. She underwent three treatments for pelvic pain; therapy started in the second year following her second pregnancy.

> *After my first delivery I had problems with my right hip. I primarily had trouble getting up after lying down or sitting. I was really tired and had a lot of trouble handling everyday chores. It took me six years to realize that I had developed chronic problems with my pelvis.*

Catherine, who experienced problems for a number of years after her first delivery, underwent conventional treatment throughout that time. She started my therapy program a year after her third delivery and received seven treatments for pelvic instability. She wrote the following when her third child was fifteen months old:

> *After having my first son I hobbled around with pain in my back and legs. Now, after eight years of pain and therapy, I realized that I had developed pelvic instability. Ironically, that realization occurred when no one was taking me seriously anymore and people were telling me I shouldn't exaggerate so much. In the last three months I've had more positive results than in all the years before. I have the feeling that I can live an almost*

painless, reasonably normal life. For eight years the specialists told me I had a hernia, but it turns out that's not what was causing the pain.

Francine had three treatments after the delivery of her third child. This excerpt was written when her third child was three months old:

I had problems during my last pregnancy, but I thought it was the baby pressing against my pelvis. Despite a lot of pain I kept walking and working. After the delivery the pain went away, but a week later it came back. After a month I finally called my doctor for help and was referred to Cecile for physiotherapy. The exercises she had me do really made a difference and helped a great deal more than simply resting.

Characteristics of Pelvic Dysfunction

Most women who have this syndrome report continuous pain. Sometimes the pain is sharp, sometimes burning or sore. It seems to focus in and around the pelvic area: in the lower back, the tailbone, the stomach, the sides or back of the thighs, the groin, or the pelvic bone. The pain can radiate downward into the legs, upward into the back, and even into the neck. One of the most annoying things about the pain is that it's so changeable; sometimes it is intense, yet at other times it may disappear suddenly, making the patient feel confused and unsure.

Once this syndrome develops, activities of daily living may become more difficult, including:

- turning over in bed
- standing for a long time
- sitting for a long time
- bending
- getting up from a couch or chair, especially a low one
- walking
- walking up and down stairs
- lying in the same position for a long time
- making love
- taking care of a child
- vacuuming, ironing, washing dishes, cooking

- ❑ getting into and out of a car
- ❑ driving
- ❑ bicycling
- ❑ swimming

Besides the general pain that can stem from the activities described above, other symptoms can include:

- ❑ menstrual pain
- ❑ digestive problems
- ❑ bloating
- ❑ pain while urinating or defecating
- ❑ incontinence

Test Yourself

Are your symptoms caused by pelvic instability? A patient with pregnancy-related pelvic pain due to misalignment of the pelvis may have problems with the following exercises. For easy reference, this section is reproduced at the back of the book.

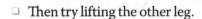 ## Test Exercise 1

- ❑ Lie down on your back and stretch out your legs.
- ❑ Try to lift one leg and then lower it.
- ❑ Then try lifting the other leg.

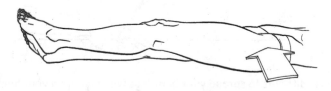

2.1. Does pushing inward against your hips make it easier to lift one leg?

If this exercise is difficult, if it hurts, or if you can't even lift your leg in this position, try to lift your leg while pressing against your hips with your hands. Use your hands to exert pressure on both sides of your hips, as if you were pushing your hips together.

If you notice that it is easier to lift your leg when you press your hands into your hips, your symptoms are probably caused by pelvic instability. If applying pressure to both sides of your hips does *not* help you to lift your leg, it may be a good idea to consult your doctor.

Test Exercise 2

Standing, try to move a light object, such as a piece of paper, forward along the floor with your foot. When pelvic instability or injury is present, this exercise will often be easier with one leg than the other.

Test Exercise 3

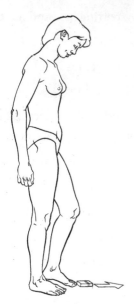

2.2. Difficult!

- ❑ Lie on your back with your legs outstretched.
- ❑ Bend your knees but keep your feet flat on the floor.
- ❑ Try to move your knees apart while keeping the sides or soles of your feet together.

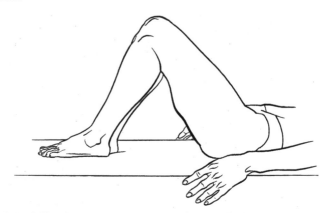

2.3. Is it difficult to spread your bent legs while lying on your back?

For someone with pelvic pain, this exercise can range from uncomfortable to extremely painful. You may experience the pain in the pubic bone or on the inside of the thighs near the groin. You may also feel pain in the lower back on either side, at one of your sacroiliac joints (due to joint compression or resistance to normal sacroiliac or lumbar movement). If you frequently experience pain in the tailbone area (the coccyx, see Figure 1.1 on page 8), this exercise may cause you to feel tension in the bottom of the pelvis.

Test Exercise 4

Sit on a hard chair for a while. If you experience pain in your tailbone, it could be caused by tension in the bottom of your pelvis. Most pelvic pain patients can only sit for a limited period of time.

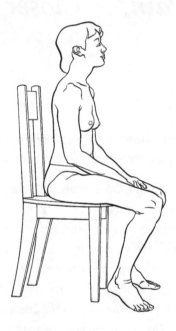

**2.4. Sitting on a hard chair without experiencing pain
is usually only possible for a short period of time.**

3

What Causes Pregnancy-Related Pelvic Pain? A Closer Look

Janice developed pelvic pain following the birth of her first child; she required three treatments approximately two months after her second pregnancy.

The delivery of my first child in 1995 was prolonged and intense; it was an assisted labor, lying down, pushing with my legs up.

The six weeks following my second delivery went badly. I definitely attempted far too much, thinking, I can do this all by myself. I really don't need any help. So, with a baby in a baby carrier and my older son (eighteen months old) in my arms, we took the train to visit Grandma, who was in intensive care. After that I took the kids to the zoo, and, of course, I was carrying far too much. I also did lots of housework soon after my delivery. There was no time to heal and recover my strength. Finally my back and pelvis gave out.

Alice had three successful treatments during her pregnancy. She gave birth to a baby girl.

Whether hormones are to blame or it had something to do with the fact that I swam so much and did gymnastics when I was young, after three months of pregnancy, I couldn't take a single step without experiencing pain.

As these two stories indicate, pregnancy-related pelvic pain can be multi-factorial (involving several different causes). This chapter examines the leading causes of the condition.

Hormones During Pregnancy

As mentioned in Chapter 1, during pregnancy, hormones ensure that all the ligaments in and around the joints become looser and more supple so that the pelvic region can be flexible during the delivery and the baby can more easily navigate the birth canal. As the ligaments become more supple, the muscles must work harder to keep the joints in place. As a result, the way you move and stand can potentially cause symptoms. However, you can also use your posture and movements to improve or prevent these symptoms.

The Pelvis Out of Balance

The pelvis is usually out of balance (asymmetrical) in patients with pelvic complaints. Typically, one of the ilia shifts against the sacrum, moving the ilium into a new position. How this displacement works probably has something to do with a woman's posture and movement patterns. For example, favoring a position in which you repeatedly put your weight primarily on one leg can promote misalignment.

To keep the pelvis in place, it's important to use several different groups of muscles: the transverse abdominal and oblique abdominal muscles; the hamstrings, gluteus maximus, and gluteus medius; and the back muscles (latissimus dorsi and multifidi). Any comprehensive therapy program to treat pelvic pain will include exercises to activate these muscles.

Let's take a closer look at some of the potential causes of this leading source of pelvic pain and dysfunction:

❑ **Poor muscle tone in the pelvic area.** One possible cause of pelvic pain is a lack of exercise in the muscles that stabilize the pelvis. For example, the gluteus medius, a strong muscle on the side of the hip, tenses when you stand firmly on one or both legs (see Figure 3.1A on the next page). However, if you frequently stand in the position shown in Figure 3.1B, the gluteus medius muscles of both hips are hardly being used, and the position of the pelvic bones is triggered to become misaligned by the failure of the stabilizing forces. A slight difference in the way weight is supported by the legs can affect the position of the pelvis. It is preferable to place your weight equally on both legs, as shown in Figure 3.1A.

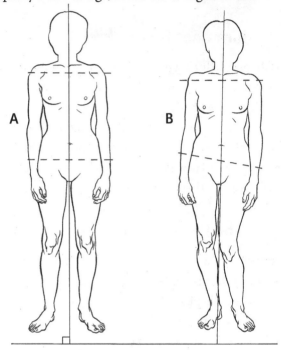

3.1. Standing postures

☐ **Poor posture.** Over the past decade scientific research has made it clear that the same muscles that correct body posture (into a position with back extended, breastbone uptilted, and shoulders low) also stabilize the pelvis and lower back.

When patients with hypermobile (very flexible) joints stand, they may overextend (overstraighten) their knees. This causes the looser ilium to rotate inward and forward, making it very difficult to use the stabilizing muscles of the pelvis. Slightly bending your knees and adjusting how your weight is distributed so that your toes are able to move freely will help your pelvis to remain stable.

Patients with pelvic pain usually sit with their legs tightly crossed or knees tightly closed, even when they drive. There is no way that you can use your stabilizing buttock or abdominal muscles if you sit like this! However, when your knees are slightly apart, stabilizing is no problem.

- ❑ **An injury affecting the joints.** Forty-five percent of pelvic pain patients report having sustained a serious fall or an accident before the pregnancy. Injuries can strain the sacroiliac joints and may cause a stiffer or more mobile joint on one side.

- ❑ **Overuse of certain muscles.** Ninety percent of pelvic pain patients report that they had previously been very active, primarily in gymnastics, swimming, horseback riding, or sailing—sports that involve frequent use of the pelvic-floor and adductor muscles.

The sacroiliac (SI) joints, located in the lower back, have large ridges and depressions that fit together like pieces in a puzzle. They are not designed for much motion. During pregnancy and delivery more motion is needed, so hormones relax the ligaments. People who were fit when they were younger have joints that are smooth and pliant. If there's a large difference in pliancy between the SI joints, using the strong adductor muscles can displace one ilium and pull it slightly forward. Often, pelvic displacement will only happen on the looser side (i.e., with one ilium).

This situation doesn't just cause back problems; it can also cause the pubic bone to twist a little, as if it were being "wrung out." Because of the way the muscles are attached, this can result in pelvic pain and a stinging sensation in the ligaments of the pelvis.

- ❑ **Heavy lifting.** I have had many patients who, as part of their job, have to do a great deal of heavy lifting or other types of strenuous manual labor. Two examples are physiotherapists and nurses. When you lift an object with your leg turned inward and your knee extended, you are asking for trouble, especially if your SI joints have been made pliable by hormonal influences. If you make this kind of movement your pelvis is not stabilized, and your pelvis can easily slip into the twisted position that can cause pelvic pain.

- ❑ **The demands of pregnancy.** Throughout pregnancy, it is difficult to use the abdominal muscles effectively to stabilize the pelvis. The abdominal muscles are stretched by the growing abdomen and by their change in function: Normally useful as stabilizers, in pregnancy they "hold" the extra weight and volume. There is no evidence that the weight of the fetus plays a role in pelvic pain. However, some evidence has shown that it is better to lose the extra weight in the year following delivery in order to have a quick recovery.

❑ **The demands of delivery.** During delivery, it's possible to displace the SI joint, especially if the mother is lying with her knees pulled up and two different people are holding a leg, each applying a different amount of pressure.

If the baby is extracted quickly (during an assisted delivery), one of the ilia may be displaced due to twisting of the pelvis. Symmetry exercises done immediately after the delivery will be able to correct the displacement (see Chapter 5). Only two aspects of the labor seem to be of significant importance in respect to the prognosis: the experience of extreme pain and the length of time a woman spends in labor. The more pain that is involved or the more time the delivery takes, the greater the risk of a slow recovery, but keep in mind that overall her prognosis is good.

Pain in the Pubic Bone

The symphysis pubis is the stiff joint connecting the pelvic bones at the front of the body below the abdomen (see Figure 1.1 on page 8). Pain at the symphysis pubis can occur when one of the pelvic ilia shifts or twists while the other stays still. As a result, the adductor muscles, which are attached to the pubic bones, sense the different position and, in an effort to correct the situation, pull hard at the bones to rotate them back into place. In response, the patient experiences a stinging, somewhat spastic pain when she tries to lift her leg.

Pain in the Tailbone

Pain in the tailbone can result from tension in the pelvic-floor muscles or from an injury. In these cases, it is important to attempt to relax the pelvic-floor muscles after rebalancing the alignment of the pelvis (see Chapters 5 and 6 for specific exercises).

Anxiety and Pain:
A Vicious Cycle

Sophie, who had two successful treatments for pelvic pain during her pregnancy, wrote to say that at thirty-eight weeks pregnant she was doing well.

> If I have pain in my pelvis (only the symphysis at this point), I lie on my back with my legs pulled up and spread wide. I also take deep breaths, rest a lot, and sleep. This has enabled me to control the pain quite well.
>
> Despite my anxiety about pelvic pain, I was able to do everything I felt like doing during my pregnancy. The result was that I was more satisfied with what I could accomplish each day, and I felt much happier and healthier.

Michelle has two daughters. Her first treatment took place six weeks after the delivery of her second child, and she had five treatments over the next eight months.

> It was good that my complaints were not so intense. It seemed normal, and normal things tend to get resolved on their own.

Tina had four successful treatments during her second pregnancy.

> I was very afraid to go through the delivery and worried about what I would feel like after it was over. I wondered if my ability to walk would be affected for the rest of my life. Now, it's as if a big stone has been lifted from my shoulders. I feel so relieved.

Ronnie was thirty-eight weeks pregnant with her first child when she was taught how to control her symptoms. In response, she elected to practice yoga during her pregnancy; she also underwent three successful treatments.

> *When I learned that I had pelvic instability, I immediately imagined the worst. I saw myself on crutches or in a wheelchair.*

All of these women, with the exception of Michelle, describe the pronounced emotional reactions they had to their pelvic pain and/or its treatment. Social worker Christine Buttinger comments on the importance of psychological factors in pain syndromes:

> *Everyone experiences anxiety and fear. Anxiety can produce positive as well as negative effects. Anxiety can prepare us to deal with a situation—fight or flight—or it can paralyze us, making us incapable of doing anything other than just waiting. When we are threatened with a real danger, such as a fire, taking immediate action is the best option. Putting the fire out or running away to call the fire department is a good idea. Sitting there paralyzed will not put the fire out.*

Women with pelvic pain are afraid to change the way they carry their bodies. Frequently the pain makes them afraid to move. Their bodies no longer function correctly. Nerves may send the wrong signals to the brain, making it difficult to know how to move. Groups of muscles designed to make other movements are called upon to keep the pelvic bones in place but may, in fact, contribute to the misalignment. The result is increasing instability and uncertainty during regular movements such as walking. This chapter looks at this chain of events, which can become a vicious, self-reinforcing cycle.

In my practice, I not only work with women who have pelvic instability; I also work with many children who have a poor sense of their bodies and how to hold them. These children sit differently and usually move more stiffly than other children. They are unsure of their bodies and are often afraid to move. Ordinary activities such as climbing stairs, standing up from sitting, or using the slide or the swings are so anxiety provoking that the children stiffen up or find it difficult to understand exactly what they should do. I work with them by observing them and then, in a playful manner, coaxing them to move more fluidly. This can help reduce the anxiety, and, with subtle guidance, ensure that the child begins to enjoy sports and physical activity.

The understanding I have gained from treating children has been useful in helping me to devise a quick, effective approach to treating my own pelvic instability symptoms. Trusting your feelings and listening to your body are necessary parts of knowing how to move, and this is true not only for children. This trust takes courage but provides satisfaction.

A lot of media attention has been given to mothers with small children who, because of pelvic instability, have wound up in wheelchairs and have had to cope with many related problems. It's not surprising that most women immediately become anxious when they get this diagnosis. The anxiety is undeserved and can, in fact, be counterproductive. When you become anxious you may attempt to hold your pelvis in the wrong way to try to "fix" things and may wind up making the symptoms worse.

Pain can also help to create the anxious feeling that one's pelvis is no longer functional. This is not true. Pain means that the pelvis is unbalanced and that there is tension in the joints and ligaments that hold these bones together. By doing the exercises in this book, you can eventually realign your bones and keep them in the right place. The pain will disappear by itself.

Insight from a Social Worker

Let's hear again from social worker Christine Buttinger:

I have spoken to several of Cecile's pelvic instability patients and have noticed how paralyzed they were by anxiety. They make comments like, "Will I irreparably damage something if I move the wrong way?" "Soon I won't be able to do anything, and I'll wind up in a wheelchair." Yet I found that these women were not generally anxious types. On the contrary, they were the type who persevered and struggled through problems on their own for a long time without asking for help.

In Anna's case (see Introduction), she experienced pain in her pelvis when she walked. She received a list of things she must not do and was asked by her physiotherapist if the pain might possibly be psychosomatic.

After a week she could no longer climb stairs. She had gotten the idea that she would permanently damage her body if she forced herself to be physically active and could wind up in a wheelchair. She was afraid to move, and she walked less and less. She was advised to "learn what her boundaries were and then do less than that." This contributed to her anxiety about being too active, damaging her body, and becoming an invalid.

After two treatments for pelvic instability, Anna could walk up a few stairs, which restored her faith in her ability to resume physical activity and to handle her delivery. Despite the positive direction that the rest of her pregnancy took, she experienced an intense delivery in which her pelvic bones were once more displaced. Although she made a rapid recovery following her delivery, her anxiety about undertaking a second pregnancy lingered. A couple of years ago I met her again. She had delivered a second baby and was very pleased that pregnancy, delivery, and recovery had gone well.

Jackie developed symptoms during her pregnancy that persisted for four years. She lived in a second-floor apartment and could only descend the stairs if she was sitting. Eventually she could only walk with crutches. She underwent physiotherapy for a year and a half with no positive results. The advice she got was "rest, rest, and more rest." Although she was employed as a doctor's assistant, she soon found she could not work and wound up on unemployment.

During these years, she often became angry or depressed because her symptoms were painful, they were severely limiting her life, and her condition had not responded to treatment. She was also anxious—anxious about becoming pregnant again and anxious about her work situation. She looked healthy, and she worried that others might assume she was just trying to get out of working.

She began to try to address the pelvic instability and to learn what she could do to prevent the pain. Once the pain began to subside, she became more physically and emotionally stable. She was planning another pregnancy and once more trusted her body and the future.

Susan's symptoms started in the fourth month of her first pregnancy, and they occurred primarily in her tailbone. She functioned and even managed to undergo a Caesarean section while enduring these symptoms. Later, when she developed more symptoms and was evaluated, the X rays showed she had a double hernia.

Although she had an operation for the hernia, the symptoms in her tailbone remained. More physiotherapy could not determine the source of the problem. She wanted to have a second child but she was anxiety ridden. She wondered how a second pregnancy would go. Her gynecologist referred her to Cecile when she became pregnant again. Later in her pregnancy, although she was having some problems associated with gaining weight, she was doing generally well because she knew what the problem was and what she had to do to make the pain go away. Her fear of potentially painful physical activity had been transformed into the reassurance that movement is what will make the pain go away.

Breaking the Cycle

In response to the pain of pelvic instability, patients often falsely assume that they should be less physically active. One's natural inclination is to go easy on oneself. Advice frequently reinforces this notion: "Watch out, be careful, rest a lot, and only move when you have to." However, this approach can lead to reduced motion and inactivity, which can result in weakness, muscle tension, and cramps, culminating in a vicious cycle (see Figure 4.1).

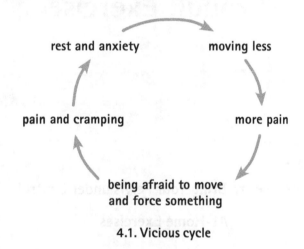

4.1. Vicious cycle

Women like Michelle, who are less anxious, typically respond well to treatment. It seems that women can be helped by focusing attention on such questions as:

- ❑ How long have these symptoms lasted?
- ❑ When did the symptoms become worse (for example, during menstruation)?
- ❑ What is "normal" or to be expected in such a situation?

When the vicious cycle is broken, recovery can begin. Anxiety lessens at the moment when women know they can do something about the pain and when they realize that exercises and movement can help alleviate it.

PART II

Relieving Pelvic Pain Through Exercise

Exercises to Bring Your Pelvis under Control

At-Home Exercises

Exercises to Bring
Your Pelvis under Control

During her pregnancy, Miranda had five treatments for pelvic instability, which effectively corrected her condition.

> *I felt freed because the exercises helped improve my posture so much. Instead of wobbling around as if I were ancient, I was able to enjoy the last months of my pregnancy and the months after the delivery.*

Tina, whom you met in the last chapter, wrote me the following note two months after her baby was delivered:

> *I went to Cecile's office with a pelvic sling and a pair of crutches, and I came home without them. My husband asked if I had been to a miracle worker. He could not believe his eyes. Before, I had asked for help doing the housework, but now I don't need it anymore. Not that my home is spotless, but at least I can do almost everything again, thanks to the exercises. Just when all was going very well, I placed my fussy baby on my knee and then lifted him. This foolishness cost me, but after more therapy everything improved again.*

Joanna, who had three treatments during her pregnancy, wrote the following when her daughter was six months old:

> *When I attempted to do too much and didn't do my exercises faithfully every day, the symptoms really bothered me, but once I did the exercises*

for even just a few minutes, I felt better. I know it sounds unbelievable, but it's true.

Catherine had seven treatments; she had endured problems since her first delivery eight years previously, for which she'd received years of treatments. She wrote to me fifteen months after she had her third child:

I never thought that I would have less pain or that one day there would be no more pain—that I would be able to do the normal things in life without pain.

Karen, who had two treatments while she was pregnant, reported on her progress when her daughter was seven months old:

It was a great gift for me to feel like I had regained control over my body. I no longer felt as if I were paralyzed but felt that I could positively influence the situation. In the beginning it almost seemed as if it were a coincidence, but in retrospect I can see that the postures and exercises really did work.

This chapter outlines introductory exercises for regaining symmetry and stability in the pelvis. They can help you no matter how long your symptoms have existed. If you have had symptoms for a long time, you may need more than one treatment before you can achieve the positions and follow the exercise advice offered here. You may worry that painful movements could potentially inflict damage to your joints. Your therapist will help you to get started and to build confidence. If you walk with crutches or are in a wheelchair, it may take a while for you to get back into condition. You won't necessarily need more treatments, but you will need to exercise consistently to improve your muscle tone.

Every patient is different, of course. Sometimes, when chronic sacroiliac instability has become "entrenched," it may take more than just a few visits to a physiotherapist to set things right again. When the problem is fairly acute (recently developed), patients will frequently respond after just a few visits and implementation of a home exercise program, but if a patient has been out of alignment for a long time or if she has experienced a new stress to the area, sometimes she'll need to return to the therapist for a "tune-up." The sort of event that could necessitate a return visit may be as seemingly insignificant as a misstep, or it could occur, for example, when a patient takes up a new sport or returns to work.

In short, if you suffer from anxiety, are in a lot of pain, or have become disabled, as mentioned in the Introduction, it may be useful for you to consult with a physiotherapist for at least the first few treatment sessions. Take this book with you to your appointment; the therapist will know what to do. I have received many enthusiastic letters telling of successful treatment by therapists who simply followed the instructions in this book. Be aware that, in the early stages of treatment, consultation with a trained physiotherapist can help enormously to get you started and to build your confidence.

If you've only had symptoms for a little while or if the symptoms are not serious, there's a chance that you may not need any therapy. Reading and following the advice in this book may suffice. Applying pressure to certain points, as illustrated in Figure 5.1, can alleviate pain in the back, pelvis, or tailbone.

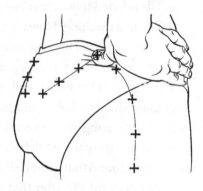

5.1. Pressure points

Personalizing the Exercises

Here are some pointers for making the most of the program provided in this book:

1. Be sure to track your progress and to take note of and be happy with every step forward you make. Compare where you are now with where you were a few weeks earlier. Note any advances in a journal—for example, the first time you can once again perform a particular movement or task. The pain may return, perhaps in a diminished way or in another location. Don't be alarmed; just repeat the exercises.

2. Take the time to make the exercises your own. Try to give your exercise regimen a daily rhythm. For instance, do your exercises every evening at

7:30 P.M. while watching a light television program or listening to your favorite music. This is your time and you want to make the most of it.

3. The symmetry and stabilization exercises outlined in this chapter are the most important; they are the ones you really have to master if you want to get rid of your symptoms. Perform the stabilization exercise whenever you can, at your own tempo. You can perform both types of exercises throughout your pregnancy, right after your delivery, or whenever you're experiencing pain.

Good luck!

Symmetry Exercise

I'd like to share with you how I developed these exercises. I taught yoga weekly. When I became pregnant, I continued teaching. However, as my pregnancy progressed, I experienced a great deal of pain. One day, during my sixth month, I had to catch a running child at the school where I worked as a physical therapist. It was a mistake: Immediately afterward I couldn't walk any farther. Still, I was determined to teach my yoga class and decided to join the group in exercising. In order to get control over the pain, during every exercise I let my knees spread apart and my thighs turn out. Despite the pain, it felt better, so I kept going.

At a certain point in the session I found that I could sit on the floor in a cross-legged "tailor's" position without discomfort. After that exercise I also noticed that my mobility was much improved—I could easily walk without pain. I realized that this position—or something similar—was key in reestablishing symmetry in my pelvic area.

I developed exercises and did them every day as a security measure to avoid the return of pain (in case something in my pelvis might again become displaced). My midwives were amazed, because the patients they knew with pelvic instability had become less and less mobile during their pregnancies. They were amazed to see me running up the stairs, because the last time they had seen me I was dragging myself up, clinging to the railing.

Again, begin with this first exercise and work though the exercises in this chapter in the order in which they are presented. The first exercise is very important because it provides the basis for all of the exercises that follow. Only after your hip muscles become flexible enough to allow your legs to move apart as described below does it make any sense to proceed with the later exercises.

To perform the initial exercise:

❑ Lie on your back with your knees bent, legs together, and feet together and flat on the floor (see Figure 5.2A).

❑ Slowly spread your knees apart until they are as far apart as possible without causing you discomfort (see Figure 5.2B).

❑ Place the soles of your feet against each other. Mentally release and relax any tension or resistance in your hip joints.

❑ If this exercise is too painful, do it—gently—with the help of a partner or a therapist (see Figure 5.2C). The person who helps you should sit at the end of your feet and hold his or her hands on your knees. Applying light pressure with the fingertips, your helper or therapist opens your knees outward toward the floor, moving steadily and surely in a clean line. *Note:* The helper must follow the direction of the arrows, moving the knees not just downward, but also away from the helper.

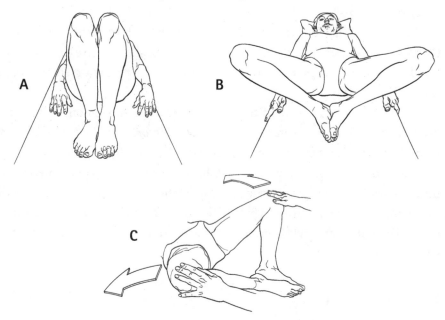

5.2A–C. Symmetry exercise

In assisting most women, a slow downward movement is easiest; for others, gently bouncing the knees one or two inches up and down in an alternating pattern (left down, right down, left down, etc.), using small, quick movements, helps to increase the stretch and overcome resistance. It may help for the woman to rhythmically tense and relax her buttock muscles (together or alternating) when the knees are almost down.

Some patients with low-back pain experience less pain with this type of exercise if they place their hands or a small pad beneath the lower back. After doing the exercise regularly for a while, this support will no longer be needed.

If the joints in your pelvis are in the right position, you will be able to move your legs flexibly and independently of each other. The right and left legs should be able to lower by the same amount; the right leg should be able to turn as far out as the left—and vice versa—when you are lying down. If this is not the case, then you want to keep trying until you can achieve this aim. Your goal here is to restore balance and symmetry to your body's structure—to improve your ability to function.

Muscles pulling on the pelvic bones can cause pain. As soon as the muscles relax, the pain will diminish. It is not always possible to move one's knees apart without pain in the lower back. However, once you can accomplish this—with or without help—the next time you do it, it will hurt a lot less.

Moving your legs back to the starting position can hurt in the beginning, but this also gets easier with repetition. At the end of the exercise, it usually feels good to move both legs down and up rhythmically. Try it yourself, or ask your therapist to assist you.

Take your time. Don't stop the exercise until this movement feels normal. This might take ten or even twenty minutes. *Important:* This exercise diminishes the muscular tension within the pelvis and gives the pelvic joints freedom to return to their original position. Stabilizing in this original position is needed immediately after completing the exercise. Stabilize as follows: Before standing up again, tighten your buttocks four of five times until doing so doesn't hurt any more. Then lift your pelvis from the floor a few times (like a bridge) until it feels easy to do so.

Symptoms

When you first perform this exercise, your legs may begin to tremble because the tension in your inner thigh muscles has suddenly changed. This is not a sign of anything serious. Relax your legs and let your knees fall apart loosely. Then simultaneously move both legs slightly sideways, first to one side and then the other, repeating a few times. Or stretch your legs, and the trembling will disappear.

Another concern sometimes expressed by clients is a fear of breaking the pubic bone; please know that this is impossible. The pubic symphysis is not a bone but a joint of fibrous cartilage that connects the pelvic bones in the front of the body. It is somewhat pliable. Over the past ten years, I have treated many, many women with this particular exercise and no one has ever been injured by it.

If you move carefully and let gravity do its work by relaxing your legs, nothing can happen that would damage your pelvis.

Making Progress

This symmetry exercise will restore the proper alignment of your pelvis by shifting the pelvic bones into a better position and restoring the function of the sacroiliac (SI) joints in your lower back. When that occurs, your pelvis will again be aligned!

Until your pelvis is stable and the muscle tone restored, you will have to keep repeating this exercise. Whenever you experience pain in your pelvis, you can do this exercise. Even after your symptoms are gone, you can continue to do this exercise. I still do it now and then as a preventive measure. I lie in this position until I sense that my legs are even; it really feels good.

Stabilization Exercise

I also developed the following stabilization exercise when I was very pregnant. I overdid it one day when I was running after a little one. That evening I experienced an intense pain in my pelvic area. Lying on my back, I found that I was unable to lift my right leg even an inch off the floor. However, it helped a little if I pressed my hands inward against my hips, as described in Chapter 2. I decided to try relaxing and exercising those muscles in warm water, so I hobbled to the bath. Once in the tub I exercised until I could lift my leg quite high without the help of my hands. When I got out of the bath, I found that the pain had gone.

What had happened in the bathtub? I later discovered the answer during a seminar in which I saw a demonstration of Vojta therapy. This approach uses the body's pressure points and weight shifting to make it easier to move. By applying pressure to a particular point for a sustained period of time, a predictable muscle reaction is provoked.

I was sitting in the bath with my heels pressed against the edge of the tub (I had to sit this way to be able to fit in the tub). I discovered that when I wanted to lift my right leg, I could do so by pushing my left heel into the edge of the tub. By pressing my left heel against a stationary surface, I set a chain of motion into play whereby the muscles stabilized my pelvis and I could raise my right leg.

Although I "discovered" this exercise while seated in the bathtub, what I describe here is a version that is done while standing (see Figure 5.3).

- ❑ Stand with your feet about hip-width apart. Lift your breastbone up toward the ceiling and relax your shoulders. Bend your knees slightly and place your weight on your heels until you no longer feel tension in your back muscles. You should be able to wiggle your toes.

- ❑ Put your weight on your left foot without bending your knees further.

- ❑ With a powerful push of your left heel, shift your body weight back to the center; you can feel that your weight is equally distributed between both legs. Stop for a moment.

- ❑ Then put your weight on your right foot, and push down into the heel. Again, you can feel your body weight shift back toward the center so that it is equally distributed. Stop there, and then repeat the exercise several times on both sides. Stop in the center every time; it is important that you learn to stand with weight spread evenly between both feet.

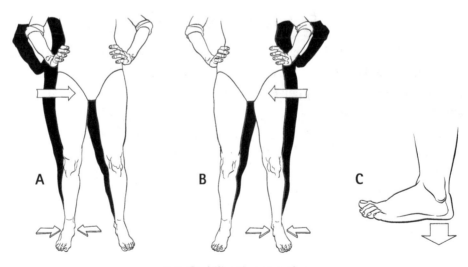

5.3. Stabilization exercise
A and B. With knees slightly bent, forcefully push your heel into the ground, shifting your weight so that it's evenly distributed between both legs; do this first on one leg then the other, stopping between repetitions to sense what it feels like to have your weight balanced.
C. Toes free, the heel pushes downward.

This exercise involves just a small movement in which you gently but firmly shift your weight from the heel and side of the foot back to the middle. *Important:* By repeating this exercise frequently, you will be able to correct any tendency to overload one side of your body, which will enable you to stabilize your pelvis in a more symmetrical position.

Repeat this exercise often—anytime you stand, wherever you are. Eventually, a reflex will be established: At the moment that your weight rests on one leg, your body will automatically push it back to center again. In this way you can prevent yourself from ever again standing with all your weight resting on one leg. I always feel that this is the most important exercise of the program; you can do it anywhere and make a habit of "safe" standing. Safe standing enhances a good walking pattern and prevents back, knee, ankle, and foot dysfunction.

If the exercise is painful, wait a couple of days and then try it again.

When I looked at myself in the mirror, I noticed that I had changed the preference of placing my weight primarily on my shorter left leg to standing on my longer right leg, which made the angle of my pelvis more crooked than ever. Noting the lack of balance in my posture, I realized I had performed this exercise only with my left leg, so afterward I did it with both legs. As I practiced this exercise I could feel which muscles were involved in my pelvic dysfunction. The muscle pain occurred on either side of my hips and directly behind them. Until that time I had not realized how weak those muscles were.

For the next week I repeated the exercise whenever I got the chance. Perhaps a thousand times a day, I made this little effort to strengthen the stabilizing muscles of my pelvis. I did the exercise everywhere—whether I was waiting in line at the supermarket, at work, or washing dishes at home. In the evening I would do the symmetry exercises, lying with my knees apart until my pelvis felt symmetrical. I paid close attention to my posture while sitting, standing, and lying on my side. I never again overextended my knees, and my ordinary posture improved greatly.

Now I do these exercises without thinking. I correct and stabilize my posture automatically. I never sit primly with my knees together the way I used to. I have adopted a much more relaxed posture. In the last five years I have become a manual therapist, which requires much more heavy lifting and vigorous movement than regular physiotherapy. It took me a couple of years of weekly yoga and fitness workouts to become strong enough to be able to perform this manual work. I feel satisfied with my body, even though it has sometimes let me down. Since I discovered these stabilization exercises, everything is going very well.

6

At-Home Exercises

Adrienne had two successful treatments two weeks before delivering her second child. When she wrote the following, her baby was four months old:

> *The last delivery went well. I got a lot out of the exercises. After the delivery, I still had some pain if I did too much housework or walked or biked too much. The first months after the baby's birth also went well. However, I had problems in certain situations; for example, if I sat in the same position for a long time, when I fed the baby on the bed, and when I gave him a bath. Generally, the exercises have helped. But when I forget to do them regularly I am overwhelmed with pelvic pain.*

There are many exercises you can use to build endurance and make your body strong again. Those presented in the last chapter are only a starting point (but a crucial one). Before participating in other forms of exercise or sports, it is advised that you practice the whole program until every exercise feels easy and you feel strong again. Here are a few general pointers regarding your exercise program:

❑ While you are pregnant, to prevent a separation of the abdominal muscles (diastasis), do *not* do the abdominal exercises shown in Figure 6.2 on page 39. It is alright to gently train the oblique and transverse abdominals during pregnancy. Doing the stabilization exercise presented in Chapter 5 adequately trains these muscles.

❑ Whereas the symmetry and stabilization exercises outlined in Chapter 5 can be done immediately after delivery, wait to begin the exercises presented in this chapter until you have resumed your normal daily activities and feel comfortable being physically active.

❑ Athletic activity in the first two years after delivery should feel easy; repetition of normal movements is more important than gaining strength.

❑ Stick to the prescribed order of the exercises.

❑ Exercise on a regular basis. Do the exercises as often and as many times as feels comfortable, even every day if you wish.

❑ Don't postpone your workouts.

❑ Don't push yourself. Remember that it generally takes most women about nine months (but often up to two years) after delivery before they feel completely normal again. Know that every now and then it's okay to take a break.

The exercises presented in this chapter are a great place to start. If you succeed in doing all the exercises and your pain is reduced, it's time to resume working out or playing sports. Wait until your baby is at least a month old before you start playing sports, and do not overdo things when you exercise or play sports. Choose an activity that you enjoy, and use it to increase your stamina.

Here's a simple exercise to try after playing sports or attending a childbirth class: Lie on the ground with your hips and knees bent, feet in the air, and legs spread apart. This stretch can help to prevent lower-back and pelvic pain.

Exercise Program

Here are some pointers for how to perform the exercises themselves:

❑ It's important to steady your pelvis as you exercise, for example, by sitting in the tailor's position cross-legged on the floor. Avoid exercising on a bed unless it is very firm.

❑ Breathe calmly during the exercises.

❑ After completing them, it can feel good to gently stretch your muscles while you're still lying down or seated.

Back Muscles

❑ This posture can be done whenever you are in a seated position, whether you are driving a car, riding a bicycle, or seated on a chair. Every now and then, press your chest upward and let your shoulder blades relax and drop (see Figure 6.1A).

❑ Sitting in the tailor's position (i.e., with knees crossed) on the floor or on a very firm bed, use your hands to pull your knees back toward your hips (see Figure 6.1B). Push your chest out, and keep your shoulders low.

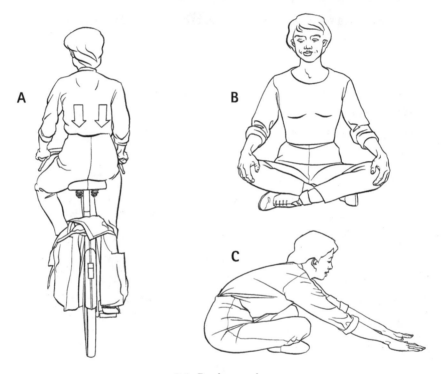

6.1. Back muscles

❑ Still in the tailor's position, stretch forward as far as you can and touch the floor in front of you while keeping your spine straight. At the same time, look up (see Figure 6.1C). Practice this stretch as often as feels necessary.

Abdominal Muscles 1

❑ Cross your arms and place your hands on opposite shoulders (see Figure 6.2A).

❑ Twist your trunk a little to the right until you feel your stomach muscles tighten; then return slowly to your starting position (see Figure 6.2B).

❑ Make the same movement to the left (see Figure 6.2C).

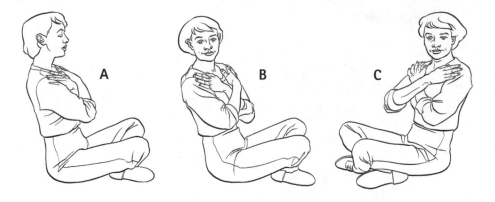

6.2. Abdominal muscles 1

Abdominal Muscles 2

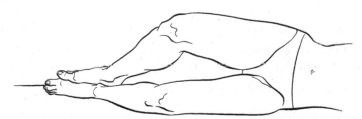

6.3. Abdominal muscles 2

❏ To exercise the muscles in your abdomen, lie on your side, and pull your navel toward the pubic bone for a short time until you sense a basic tension in your transverse (lower) abdominals. You will feel a flattening of your abdomen. Maintain this tension. Then, pushing your heels together, spread your knees about a foot apart (see Figure 6.3). Bring your knees back together and then relax your transverse abdominals. Repeat while lying on the other side.

❏ A very good exercise for training your transverse abdominal muscles (which will allow you to get better control of your pelvis) is the following: Lie on your back, and make sure your hips and knees are bent and your feet are on the mat. Pull your navel into the direction of your pubic bone and try to hold this transverse abdominal tension while simultaneously tensing one buttock for five seconds and then relaxing it for five seconds. Only when the buttock is fully relaxed should you let go of the tension in the abdominals. Repeat with the other buttock.

Spinal Twist

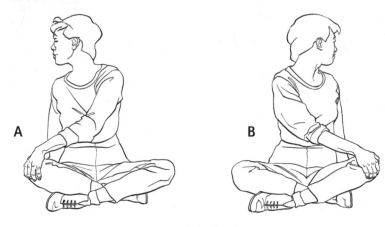

6.4. Spinal twist

- Sitting cross-legged on the floor, place your left hand on your right knee. Put your right hand behind you on the floor, with arm outstretched. Turn your head and right shoulder to the right as far as possible. Keep your chest facing forward (see Figure 6.4A).

- Reverse the position of your hands and repeat the stretch to the left (see Figure 6.4B).

Spinal Stretch

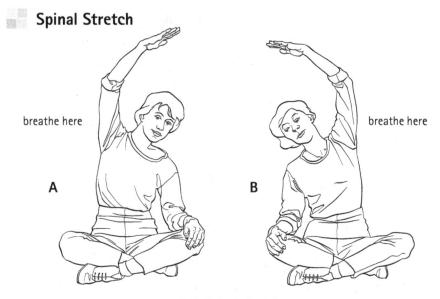

6.5. Spinal stretch

❑ From a seated position, bend slightly sideways and stretch your arm high above your head. Be sure not to bend forward at the trunk, but keep your chest elevated and your shoulders square to the front (see Figure 6.5A).

❑ Breathe in and out at the top of the move. Exhale as you bring your arm back down.

❑ Repeat to the other side (see Figure 6.5B).

Forward Stretch 1

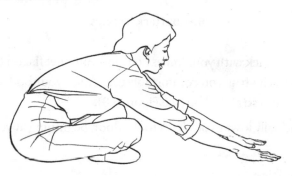

6.6. Forward stretch 1

❑ While in the tailor's position (legs crossed), calmly stretch your fingers on the floor in front of you while keeping the upper part of your spine straight (see Figure 6.6).

Forward Stretch 2

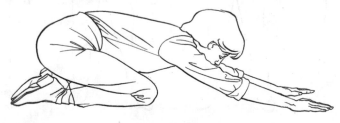

6.7. Forward stretch 2

❑ In a kneeling position, rest your buttocks on your heels with your knees apart. Move your hands forward on the floor while keeping your buttocks resting on your feet (see Figure 6.7).

■ Buttock Muscles

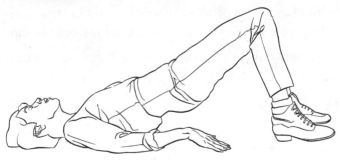

6.8. Buttock muscles

❑ Lie on your back with your knees bent and your feet flat on the floor. Raise your hips as high as you comfortably can. Align your body from knees to shoulders in a straight line (see Figure 6.8).

❑ Now gradually lower your back to the floor, beginning at your neck.

■ Coordination

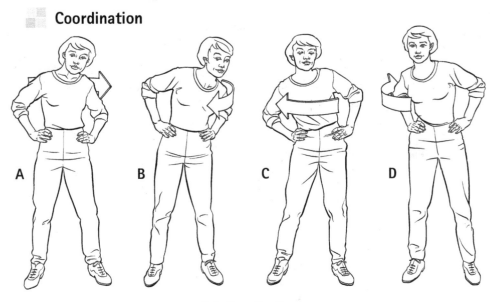

A   B   C   D

6.9. Coordination

❑ Using a small amount of motion, calmly and with concentration bend your torso to the left, to the front, to the right, and back to center (see Figures 6.9A–D). Repeat, reversing the direction.

❑ Move the top of your torso, but do not move your hips (i.e., bend at the waist).

❑ With your hands, push downward on your hipbones (ilia) throughout the exercise.

◼ Circulation and Pelvic-Floor Muscles (see text on the next page)

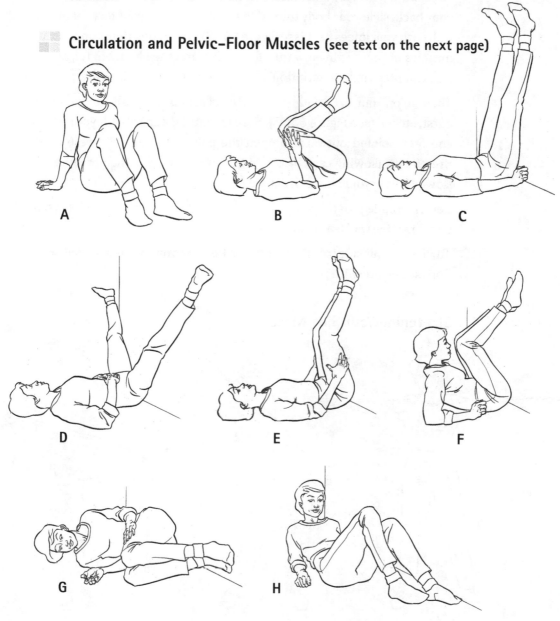

6.10. Circulation and pelvic-floor muscles

Note: During menstruation it is better to skip this exercise. There is some thought that the feet-upward position may cause a backward flow of blood, which may contribute to endometriosis.

☐ Sit facing a wall (see Figure 6.10A on the previous page). Then lie down on your back, slide your body toward the wall, and place your feet flat on the wall with your knees bent (see Figure 6.10B). In this position, contract the muscles of your vagina inward a few times, and then let them fully relax (see Chapter 8 for a description of how to do this pelvic-floor exercise).

☐ Then lie on your back with your buttocks against the wall and your legs outstretched (see Figure 6.10C). Spread your legs apart with your knees and feet pointed outward to open the pelvic area (see Figure 6.10D). Breathe in, allowing each breath to fill your abdomen. Then breathe out slowly, letting your stomach deflate.

☐ Return your legs to the middle (see Figure 6.10E). Then gently slide your feet down the wall (see Figure 6.10F).

☐ Turn onto your side (see Figure 6.10G). Resume your original seated position (see Figure 6.10H).

Stretching Your Side Muscles

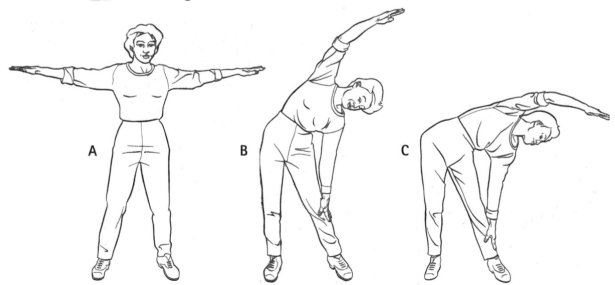

6.11. Stretching your side muscles

❏ Stand with your feet apart, knees slightly bent, and arms extended at shoulder level (see Figure 6.11A). Breathe in, pulling your stomach flat.

❏ Bending your torso to the left while keeping your hips centered and your weight evenly distributed between both legs, raise your right arm to the side and then over your head, breathing out as you stretch (see Figure 6.11B). Keep your hips, chest, and shoulders square to the front.

❏ If you can accomplish it without great discomfort, take the stretch even lower. Keeping your right arm horizontal, take two deep breaths and then inhale deeply as you return to an upright position (see Figure 6.11C).

❏ Repeat the exercise to the other side.

Exercycling in a Standing Position

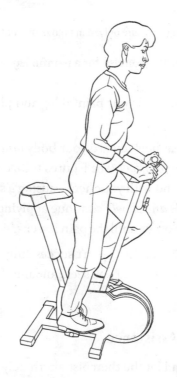

6.12. Exercycling in a standing position

❏ Once you are feeling strong again, using the exercycle while standing is a great way to further strengthen your pelvis.

Additional Symmetry Exercises

If your pelvis continues to be out of alignment, it may prove difficult to perform the symmetry exercise outlined in Chapter 5. In order to correct the alignment in your pelvis, try the following exercises:

Exercise for a Painful Leg

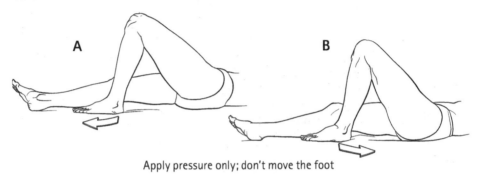

Apply pressure only; don't move the foot

6.13. Exercise for a painful leg

- ❏ Lying on your back, bend your painful leg and place the foot flat on the floor.
- ❏ Then try to push that heel toward your body and then away from it, *but don't actually move your foot* (see Figures 6.13A and B). You're applying pressure to the ground with your heel, causing a subtle movement in the pelvis. *Rhythmically and slowly* continue applying pressure in one direction and then in the other until the pain lessens.

Important note: If this exercise doesn't successfully relieve the pain within ten minutes, it is recommended that you seek guidance from a manual therapist or chiropractor.

Exercising with Assistance

- ❏ Lie on your side, and let the therapist alternately resist the bending (see Figure 6.14A) and extending (see Figure 6.14B) of your upper knee and, at the same time, adjust your ilium.

You can do a variation of this exercise on your own by following the instructions for the next exercise.

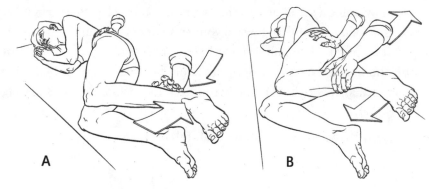

6.14. Exercising with the assistance of your therapist

▨ Relieving a "Locked" Pelvis (see text on the next page)

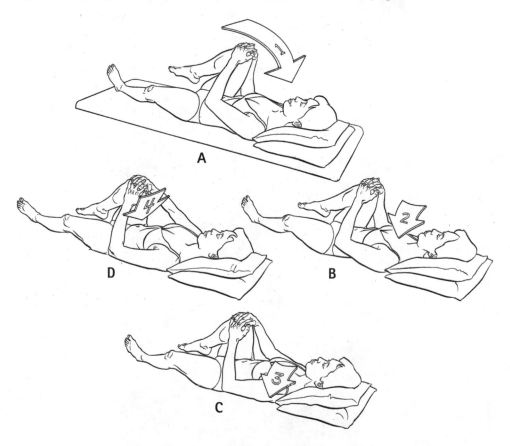

6.15. What to do if your pelvis feels locked

❑ Begin by doing a series of stretches with the painful leg. Start by pulling the knee of the painful leg toward your shoulder (see Figure 6.15A on the previous page). Then pull it toward your chest (see Figure 6.15B). Now pull the knee toward your opposite shoulder (see Figure 6.15C). Then push your knee with both hands in the direction of your buttocks (see Figure 6.15D).

❑ Repeat with the other (usually less painful) leg.

PART III

Daily Activities

Listen to Your Body

Sitting, Standing, and Lying Down

Pointers for Everyday Activities

7

Listen to Your Body

Karen, who received two treatments during her pregnancy, wrote to me when her daughter was seven months old:

About a week after the delivery, I was in pain. The pain remained for several weeks, but after I rested and made sure to move very carefully, it went away. At that point I began doing pelvic-floor exercises more often, which really helped.

Joanna, whom we first heard from in Chapter 5, had three treatments during her pregnancy:

What surprised me most in this program is that I had to turn my legs outward. In a previous pregnancy I was told never to do that; I was only allowed to move my legs up and down, which was the movement that caused me the most pain!

Pauline, my first pelvic patient, came to me five times. She wrote the following when her daughter was almost two:

Despite receiving physiotherapy for a year after my delivery, I was still in pain. The new exercises you gave me were quite different from those given to me by my previous physiotherapist—your exercises did not hurt. After five or six treatments I improved so much; I am almost always pain free now.

During each of my own three pregnancies, I experienced fairly intense pelvic pain. When I was pregnant for the third time and again had serious pelvic pain symptoms, I decided to seek a new solution. I wanted to go beyond the advice I had been given and what I had read, because none of the things I had heard or read had made my pregnancies or deliveries any easier.

After the delivery of my second child I began to exercise to strengthen my muscles. Luckily I already knew which muscle groups I had to strengthen to stabilize my pelvis. Only at that point did I start to mend and did the pain begin to disappear. However, despite that success, it still took me two years after the birth of my second child to be able to take part in sports again.

Finding Self-Help Techniques That Work for You

When I became pregnant for the third time, I arranged my pregnancy leave and prepared for the worst. During my first two pregnancies I'd had months when I could not walk, so my doctor and my midwife assumed that I might be in a wheelchair by my sixth month. At only nineteen weeks pregnant, I could see crutches and a wheelchair in my immediate future. That is when I started to think seriously about the problem and to listen to my body. Here are some strategies I came up with at that time:

1. *Balancing rest with activity.* I began to wonder why I should rest so much when it had not helped during my first two pregnancies. I decided not to rest for more than an hour at a time during the day. Rather than lying in bed, I rested on the couch, half sitting up, so that my muscles wouldn't completely relax. I knew that my pelvis was very lax, so my muscles would have to supply some stability for me to be able to get up again.

   By resting on the couch while reading or listening to nice background music, I could get the rest I needed. Lying peacefully and breathing deeply helped provide emotional relaxation.

2. *Taking time to stretch before standing.* I decided to stretch my muscles before standing. Taking a deep breath, I stretched out my arms and tightened my buttocks. Then I pulled in the bottom of my pelvis (i.e., performed a pelvic-floor contraction, otherwise known as a Kegel exercise; see Chapter 8). At that point I stood up.

3. *Using posture to stabilize the body.* I noticed that I had the hardest time walking after I had been sitting with my knees close together very primly, the way I had been taught to do as a young girl. I also began to notice that my lower back would become tense and I had to keep changing the

position of my legs to continue sitting this way. I couldn't understand why I was given the advice to hold my thighs tightly together. I believed that my problems associated with pelvic instability arose because of the SI joints in the lower back. Wasn't the pain in the area of the pubic bone also primarily the result of instability in the back of the pelvis?

I wondered if sitting with my knees slightly apart might help. I soon realized that this is a much more stable way to sit because your base is a triangular shape. You will also find that you sit much more securely if your feet are placed flat on the floor or if you put them up on a footstool. I experimented with different sitting postures—for example, I sat with my knees as far apart as possible in order to find out whether my pain would subside or worsen afterwards. The pain subsided.

4. *Becoming attuned to one's body.* I had become curious about the puzzle presented by pelvic problems and decided to focus my efforts on figuring it out. I decided to walk without aids for as long as possible.

As a result of implementing these self-help strategies and doing my exercises faithfully, I had a fantastic third pregnancy. I took frequent walks until the day of my delivery and I enjoyed the days after, rejoicing in the fact that I had so little pain and that I could still move so well. Six weeks after the delivery, I went back to work. I no longer have any symptoms. Even the residual problems from the earlier pregnancies and deliveries have disappeared. To this day, I continue to do my exercises.

Basic Rules

One aspect of restoring balance to your body involves unlearning old habits and postures. To avoid pelvic complaints, remember the following five things:

1. When sitting down, never hold your knees together or press them against each other.

2. While standing, place your weight evenly on both legs, with your knees slightly bent and slightly turned out.

3. Pain may be a sign that your pelvis is not balanced. Once your normal symmetry and mobility are restored, the pain will disappear.

4. Do not be afraid that you will break a bone if you are in pain and want to exercise. Pain means the ligaments are strained, which interferes with

your sense of how to move properly. Exercise will restore the tone in your muscles and the "position sense" in your joints, supporting the correct alignment of the pelvic bones. Once the tension is removed from the muscles and ligaments, the pain will disappear.

5. Listen to your body.

8

Sitting, Standing, and Lying Down

Lisa, who had two treatments, now has three children, the youngest a twelve-month-old daughter.

> I remember very well as a child learning that it was not nice for girls to sit with their legs apart. My aunt was very relaxed about how she sat, but my sisters and I were ashamed of her and giggled about it. We would never do that! We definitely wouldn't sit like that if we were wearing short skirts, which was often the case.
>
> We learned, as did our friends, to walk in the "proper" way, with our knees close together, to be attractive and yet "decent." If we had to pick something up from the ground, we had to do it with our knees together (especially if our skirts were too short), which is not easy. It was a struggle to assume these awkward postures. It's odd that one never unlearns this curious way of holding oneself.

Recently, I spoke to a seventy-year-old acquaintance about the way she sat with her knees neatly together. Surprised, she asked me how she should be sitting. When I told her about sitting in a more relaxed way, she blurted out, "Yes, but you're not supposed to sit that way." Unfortunately, she has a long history of pelvic complaints. She has experienced low-back pain for years (ever since her last pregnancy). Recently, she had five treatments for her back and pelvis with a chiropractor before she could stand up straight and walk comfortably again. Even so, she regularly did "forbidden" movements (e.g., bending over with straight knees) and afterwards experienced some problems. She almost always experiences some back pain, despite exercising her abdominal muscles regularly. That pain could be the result of her lifelong habits and posture. (Sitting with knees primly closed seems to be emphasized much more in some families and in certain cultures than in others.)

Sitting

When one or both of the SI joints in your lower back are more pliant than average (as they are during pregnancy), they may start to move slightly out of alignment when you press your knees together (see Figure 8.1A). The ilia may move apart slightly in your back, behind the sacrum, and move closer together at the symphysis joint. (The pubic symphysis is a flexible seam of cartilage that is located at the center of the pelvic area, below the abdomen and above the vagina; it joins the two ilia in the front. See Figure 1.1 on page 8.) Pressing your knees together is not a good idea because the symphysis becomes weakened and swollen during pregnancy, so it feels as if you were pushing against a painful joint. The sensation can be compared to a bruise on a finger. Naturally, bending it will hurt. If you feel you must sit with legs crossed, allow the legs to be more relaxed and the knees to turn outward, as in Figure 8.1B. Crossing the legs unbalances

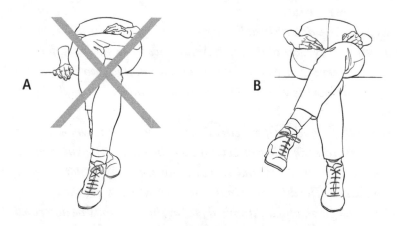

8.1. Sitting with legs crossed
A. Wrong: Knees turned inward. B. Slightly better: Knees turned outward

your pelvis, but this will not cause any painful misalignment. Asymmetry in leg or arm movement or posture is not the cause of pain; it is natural, for example, to have a dominant hand and leg.

It is best to sit in a position in which your hip muscles are relaxed. This way, the sacroiliac joint is not under any kind of pressure. To attain this position the back of your chair should recline a little bit or your hips should be a little higher than your knees so you can hold your legs comfortably down and apart with your thighs turned outward. You may cross your feet under your chair or sit at the front of your seat to achieve this posture. If you sit this way and keep your back straight, you won't look odd. It's just a matter of getting used to it. Figure 8.2 on the following page illustrates several good sitting postures.

Why do women, at least in some cultures, sit differently than men do? Why do many women whom I treat in my practice sit with their knees pressed together, even if it causes them pain and affects the way they walk? I have thought a lot about these questions in the last few years. As your pregnancy advances into the later months, the advantages of a more open, relaxed posture are really noticeable. When pregnant women sit with their legs apart, the stomach fits more easily between the legs.

Researchers have pointed out that not only are men's bone structures different from women's, but their movement patterns also differ (Van Gelder 1997):

There's a marked difference in sitting postures: men generally sit with their legs apart while women sit with their legs close together, no matter what clothing they are wearing.

Is this difference determined by men's anatomy, as is the difference in walking patterns? No, absolutely not! Anatomically seen, this difference in posture is rather strange because men and woman are both most stable when the support is widest, with legs apart and feet turned slightly outward....

The most tiring and least practical [seated] position is when the feet are placed next to each other directly under the knees. The knees naturally want to turn outward and standing up this way is not possible without wobbling. The difference in the sitting posture is not the result of genetic, physiological, and anatomical factors, but can only be described as cultural. To sum this up, only the sitting posture of a man is determined by functional anatomy; [a woman's] is determined by cultural norms.

Sitting More Comfortably

❑ Sit with your knees apart and turned out.

❑ Sit in positions that relax your lower back while it remains supported, perhaps with a cushion. Or sit upright when the back is not supported.

❑ Stretch your hips by sitting closer to the edge of your seat, leaning back, and resting your weight against the back of the chair (see Figure 8.2A).

❑ You can also stretch your hips by sitting high enough so that your knees are lower than your hips (see Figures 8.2B and C) or by crossing your feet under your chair. The important thing is to create a position where your belly is some distance from your thighs.

❑ Sit cross-legged in the tailor position (see Figure 8.2E).

❑ Use a ball cushion (see below).

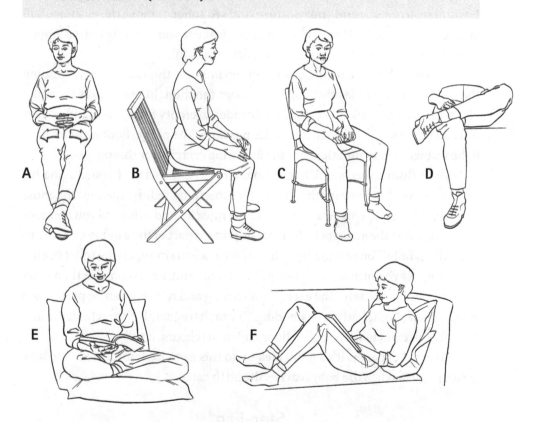

8.2. Good postures for sitting
A. Sitting with legs crossed and outstretched. B. Good seated posture.
C. Minimizing pain in the tailbone with a ball cushion. D. Relaxed sitting posture.
E. Cross-legged in the tailor's position. F. A good posture for resting.

Pelvic-Floor Muscles

Pain in your tailbone when you sit could be caused by tension in the pelvic-floor muscles. This may be remedied by stretching your hips, pushing your legs downward away from your torso (see box for specific sitting postures), and letting your vaginal muscles relax as much as possible—that is, allowing them to expand downward or outward, as happens naturally when you inhale. Once the tailbone is released, the pain will disappear.

Another practical idea is to sit on a ball cushion, positioned so that your tailbone is free (see Figure 8.2C on the previous page). A ball cushion is easy to sit on, and it keeps you in a good position. When you use it, you tend to develop active stomach and back muscles over time as a result of trying to maintain your balance. Until endurance has built up, however, sitting on a ball cushion may actually promote slumping once you become fatigued. Pay attention to your body. If you start to fatigue and your posture starts to suffer, remove the cushion. Ball cushions are available through the Internet; just use your favorite search engine to find retailers. The 33-centimeter size fits most adult females.

If you have become incontinent, you can improve this condition by training the pelvic-floor muscles that control bladder function. In most cases the muscles are too tight; they don't allow the bladder to empty fully. The bladder stays full and then overflows when it is under pressure. The pelvic-floor muscles have to be trained in coordination; use the following exercise for this purpose.

Pelvic-floor exercise: While sitting, tense the muscles of your vagina inward as if you were attempting to clench something tightly; then let the muscles relax. Inhale deeply when you relax the muscles and exhale as you contract them. Relaxing the muscles is the most important part of the exercise; be sure to relax them fully. You can practice this exercise when sitting on the toilet during urination. As you urinate, try to stop the flow of urine for a moment; then relax the muscles completely. The exercise of tensing and relaxing can be performed at any time, whether sitting or standing. Repeat it frequently throughout the day, focusing on clenching the pelvic floor and then relaxing it fully.

During pregnancy, it's a good idea to do this exercise faithfully so it will be easier to push when the baby reaches the birth canal.

Standing

When standing, as discussed in earlier chapters, it is important to balance your body weight to protect your lower back and SI joints. Because these joints are more vulnerable during pregnancy, exhibiting poor posture by, for example, walking with your weight thrust forward, could slide the sacrum out of its correct position. The result can be instability and painful symptoms.

If you stand properly, you can feel your lower-back muscles relax. Starting at your ankles, if you move your whole body a little forward and back, you can feel at what point the tension in your back subsides or returns. You may notice that you feel less tension in your back muscles if you place your weight on your heels rather than the balls of your feet (see Figure 8.3). This is the best standing position because your pelvis is most stable due to the slightly flexed position of your hips and knees. When you are standing, you should be able to move your toes.

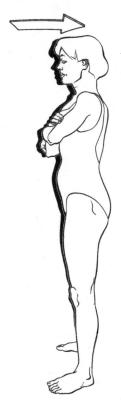

8.3. Standing

Good Standing Posture

☐ Bend your knees slightly.

☐ Stand in a way that causes the least amount of tension in your back muscles. Generally, your body will move a little bit backward, and you may feel more weight on your heels.

☐ The muscles of your thighs should be actively engaged so they seem to carry your body. When this occurs, your back muscles can relax, your transverse abdominal muscles are engaged, and you acquire a good, stable, relaxed posture.

☐ Distribute your weight evenly upon both legs.

☐ Point your toes outward a little.

This posture may feel unnatural in the beginning, but if you look in the mirror you'll see that it looks quite normal.

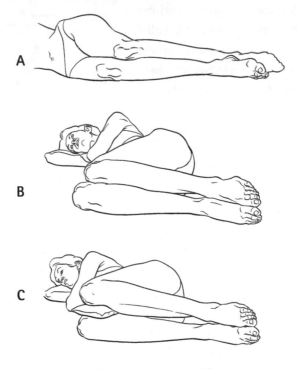

8.4. Lying on your side

Lying Down

If it feels comfortable to do so, there's no reason not to lie on your back. Lying on your stomach should not cause problems either. This will be easier after delivery, once you no longer have a big stomach and your pelvis has returned to normal. Lying on your side is also possible, but if you do so, remember to either position your upper hip a little to the rear, or move your upper leg slightly behind the lower leg, so that your SI joints are neatly positioned in a neutral, comfortable way (see Figures 8.4A and B). Placing a cushion between your knees may also be helpful (see Figure 8.4C).

Pointers for Everyday Activities

Sophie, whom we first heard from in Chapter 4, had two successful treatments for pelvic pain during her pregnancy. When she wrote the following, she was thirty-eight weeks pregnant:

When I'm tired and I want to lie down, I give in to that feeling. I rest on a regular basis. Every day or two I lie down in the afternoon for an hour, and I go to bed early in the evening.

Regarding posture, when I sit I spread my legs apart more, and I sit on the foundation that this position creates. When I stand up, I use both legs and try to apportion my weight evenly on both legs.

I exercise regularly and keep my legs a comfortable distance apart during everyday activities. I pay attention to my movements. For example, I have found a better way to turn over in bed. I rise very slowly, using my heel as support. I also wear wide, flat shoes.

Ronnie, whom you first met in Chapter 4, had three treatments during her first pregnancy, and she also practiced yoga:

Cecile assured me that with the right exercises and movements I would not have to use crutches. You would have to see my progress to believe it! It wasn't easy to remember how to carry out the different movements, but it worked. I went from having a lot of pain in my tailbone and pelvis to having only occasional pain. I now know what I can and what I can't do.

Many pelvic pain patients discover ways of moving during everyday activities that greatly aid their healing process. This chapter provides lots of pointers for performing daily activities in ways that protect the pelvic region.

In general, for the first years after delivery, we advise women to participate in sports and other activities but warn them against being overactive; we tell them to build up slowly. For the first year or two after the arrival of a new baby, remind yourself that delivery occurred only a short while ago; you will tire easily and your hormones will still be fluctuating.

Performing Daily Activities

Standing Up

Set your feet firmly on the floor, placing your hands on your thighs before you stand up (see Figures 9.1A and B). Once you are standing, put your weight on your heels and bend your knees slightly (see Figure 9.1C).

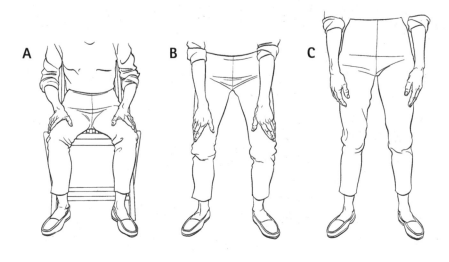

9.1. Standing up

Getting Dressed

Until your muscle tone improves, if your leg is being uncooperative try guiding it with your hands (see Figure 9.2A). If standing on one leg remains difficult, dress yourself while sitting down (see Figure 9.2B).

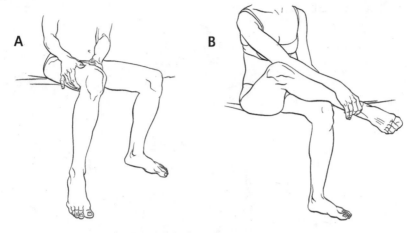

9.2. Getting dressed

Turning to One Side

When standing, turn your legs a little to the outside (see Figure 9.3A). When turning, point your toes in the direction in which you are turning (see Figure 9.3B). Maintain some distance between your knees as you turn. Stepping out with the legs spread apart is easier than taking small steps (see Figure 9.3C).

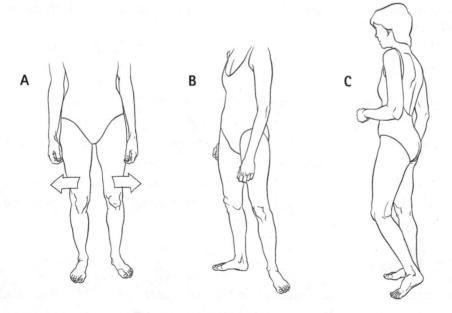

9.3. Turning to one side

Climbing Stairs

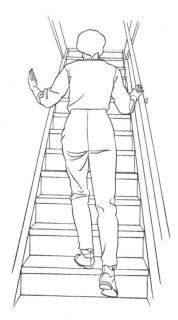

9.4 Climbing stairs

First do the stabilization exercise (see Chapter 5) and then go straight up. Do not lean heavily on available handholds such as a railing or a wall if you can help it. Just stabilize when needed. Your hands will guide you if you lightly touch the handholds.

Driving

Driving is the last in a list of movements that over time become possible to resume without causing pain. In a car it can be difficult to achieve a stable position. The constant vibration can destabilize the pelvis, and it is difficult to brace oneself against slight disturbances. Remember to keep your knees apart as you drive, and try to stop, get out of the car, and stretch your legs periodically. When using the brake, tense your buttock muscles. For more tips related to driving and getting into and out of cars see Figures 9.5A–F.

Riding a Bike

When you're riding a bicycle, keep your feet firmly on the pedals. Make sure that your foot is placed relatively perpendicular to your calf (i.e., don't point your toes, as you might in a ballet class). The bicycle seat height should be adjusted

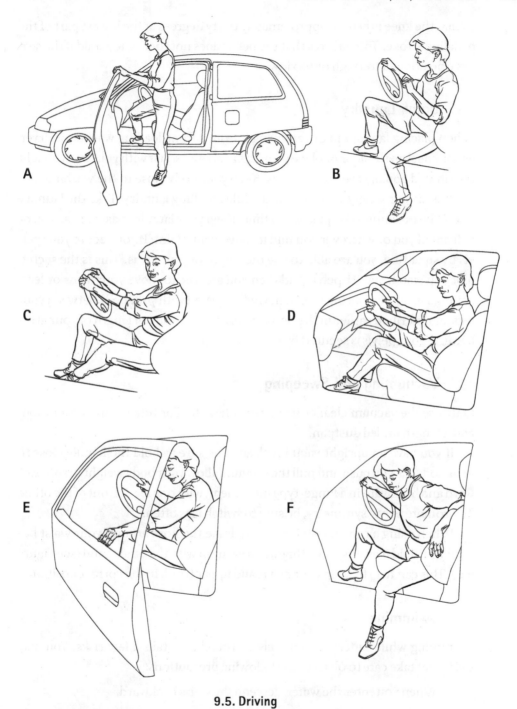

9.5. Driving

A. When getting into a car, keep your knees apart. B. Don't turn your left leg inward.
C. Next, place the left (second) leg inside the car. D. Ride with your legs apart.
E and F. Get out of the car the same way you entered it.

so that the knee is bent to approximately thirty degrees at the lowest part of the pedaling stroke. This ensures that the pelvis does not rock as it would if the seat were positioned too high or too low.

Doing Laundry

When placing laundry in or removing it from a front-loading washer or dryer, either kneel on the floor or place your legs apart and squat with your body weight distributed equally over both knees. Keep your body close to the washing machine and your weight over your feet while handling laundry. Take the laundry out of the machine a few pieces at a time. Keep your laundry basket near you or in front of you or wherever you find it convenient. (Hint: If you secure your pelvis by squatting, you are able to use the length of your arms. This is the secret; first you stabilize your pelvis and then you are free to move your arms or legs. Another example: During pregnancy, when seated with your belly between your legs, as described earlier in the book, it is safe to use the full length of your arms because your pelvis is secured by your posture.)

Vacuuming and Sweeping

Only use the vacuum cleaner if you really have to. For tidying up, use a broom and a long-handled dustpan.

If you have an upright vacuum cleaner, be sure to hold the handle close to your body. As you push and pull the vacuum, allow your body weight to shift forward and backward in a lunge-type movement, with one leg in front of the other. To promote pelvic symmetry, be sure to switch legs often.

When using a canister-style cleaner, drape the hose around your waist behind you, hold it against your thigh, and vacuum with the other hand (see Figure 9.6). This can help to keep your pelvis and upper trunk in the correct position.

Swimming

Swimming while suffering from pelvic instability entails a few risks. You may swim, but take care to observe the following precautions:

- ❑ When you enter the water, descend the stairs backward.
- ❑ When doing the breaststroke, you may have a tendency to press your legs together. If so, contract, tighten, or tense your buttocks when closing your

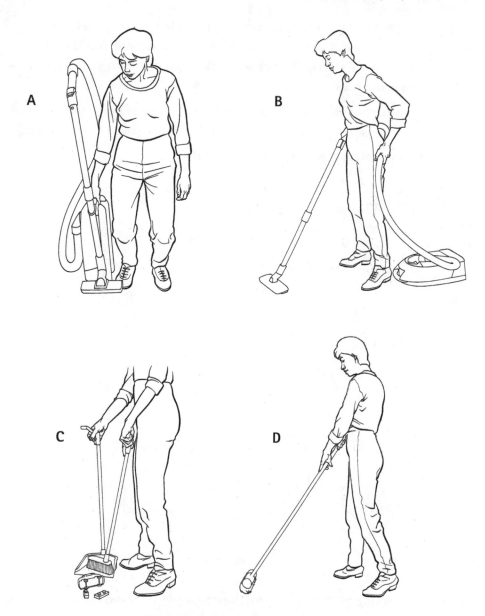

9.6. Vacuuming and sweeping
A. To pick up or put down the vacuum cleaner, let
yourself sink through your knees into a semisquatting position.
B. Place your weight on your heels and turn your knees outward.
C. To pick up small toys, use a broom and long-handled dustpan,
or get a reacher, which can be purchased at a medical supply store.
D. When using a mop or long-handled brush, turn your knees outward;
your weight should rest primarily on your heels.

legs. By doing this the movement becomes less stressful on the muscles attached to your pelvic bone and there will be less risk of pelvic pain afterward. Use of your arms in the backstroke strengthens the stabilizing muscles in your back.

❑ Stabilize your pelvis as you come out of the water by doing the stabilization exercise described in Chapter 5. Be careful to balance your weight.

❑ Be sure to wear shoes or sandals on wet floors.

Shopping

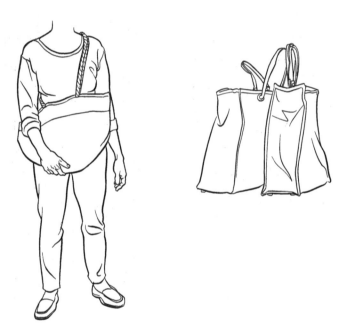

9.7. Shopping

If you are carrying a shoulder bag, put the strap over your head before filling the bag. Another option is to carry two bags of equal weight, one on each side, or to use a backpack.

Turning Over in Bed

Bending one leg, roll your body over the outstretched leg (see Figure 9.8A). Your arm starts the motion, your knee stays high, and the pelvis is lifted by tensing the upper buttock (see Figure 9.8B). Keep the foot of your top leg in place to keep your body stable until the pelvis is positioned in a side-lying position (see Figure 9.8C). Next, bend your bottom leg if you want to sit up (see Figure 9.8D). If you want to go from lying on your side to lying on your back, follow the above instructions in the reverse order. To sit up at the edge of the bed, you can lower your bent legs over the side of the bed while simultaneously pushing yourself into a sitting position with your arms.

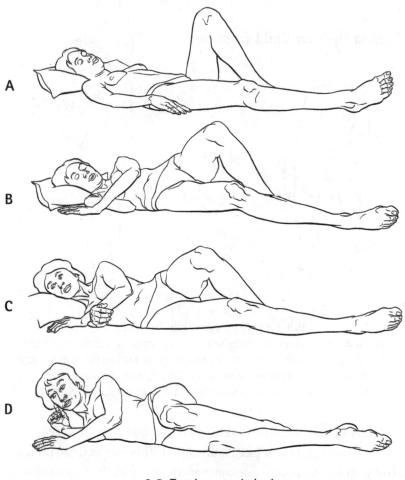

9.8. Turning over in bed

Making Love

If you are experiencing pain in your pelvic area, making love may not seem appealing. Almost none of my patients could initially make love in a normal way, sometimes not at all. However, as soon as women can painlessly perform the symmetry exercise (Chapter 5), they no longer have any problems. The only advice I would give women is that they avoid choosing any positions in which they have to place their knees together. A more open posture is definitely better. The thigh should turn outward, just as you have learned in the exercises and other activities.

Taking Care of Your Child

Picking Up Your Child from Bed

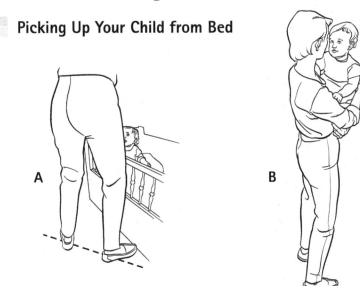

9.9. Picking up your child from bed
A. Stand diagonally in relation to the bed. Legs are turned slightly outward. Bend at the knees and hips into a semisquatting position while keeping the spine straight.
B. Position the baby as close to you as possible. Then pick the baby up and straighten your knees and hips while still keeping your back straight.

Place your feet in a slanted line in relation to the bed so your knees can move outward when you bend them (see Figure 9.9A). This way, you can lift using the strength of your legs, bending your knees and hips rather than your spine, which remains straight. This helps your pelvis to remain stabilized.

Changing Your Baby

Use the same diagonal position as the one described above when you are changing the baby's diapers on the changing table. Bend your knees, with your thighs turned outward. (Don't forget to hug the baby!)

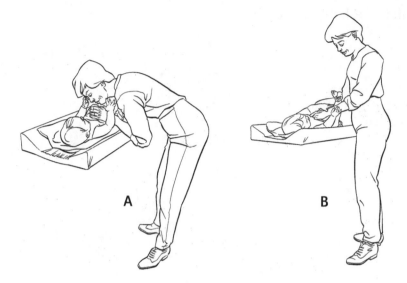

9.10. Changing your baby

A. Stand with bent knees, feet diagonal in relation to the changing table.

B. Diapers, clothes, and cleaning supplies should be placed at an easy height
for you to conveniently reach them; keep your feet turned outward.

Picking Up the Baby

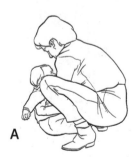 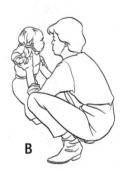 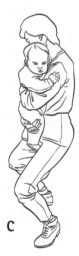

9.11. Picking up the baby

A. Don't squat for too long.

B. Keep your knees apart and your back straight.

C. Lift the baby by straightening your legs. Make lifting a supple movement.

Holding a Baby on Your Lap

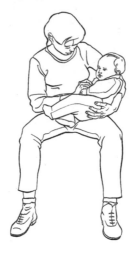

9.12. If your sitting position is stable, you can move freely.

If you choose a stable position to sit in, it's safe to have your child on your lap.

Baby Carrier

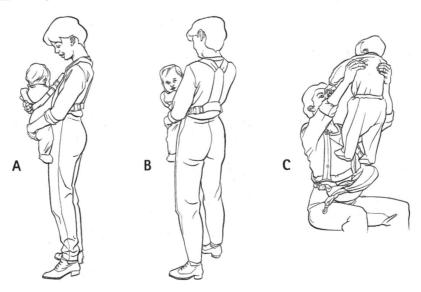

A   B   C

9.13. Baby carrier
A. A baby carrier should provide good support for your back and have straps that cross.
B. The weight of the baby adjusts your own weight backwards. This is a good thing.
C. To put your child in the carrier, sit down in a stable position with your knees apart, and then lower your baby into the carrier.

A Snugli or front-wearing baby carrier is not only a handy way to carry your baby; it can also help alleviate some of your problems. The sacrum may tilt forward when it is not properly stabilized between both ilia; this causes pain. When you're wearing a Snugli, to counteract the extra weight on the front of your body, your trunk shifts backward so that the sacrum is stabilized between the ilia. The result is better posture when walking.

When using this type of baby carrier, make sure the baby is positioned safely inside. Always check to see if the baby is breathing well. Avoid overdressing the baby, since babies cannot regulate their temperature easily. For this reason, don't use the baby carrier under your coat.

Using the Stroller

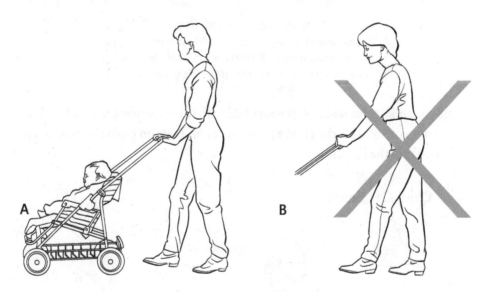

9.14. Using the stroller
A. Hold the stroller handle next to you, and keep your posture erect.
B. Avoid bending over the handle of the stroller.

When walking with a stroller, remember to keep your weight more on your heels. This will be easier if you keep the stroller near your body rather than extending your arms while pushing. By doing this you can prevent pain or discomfort caused by tension in the ligaments of the SI joints or by the overuse of the back muscles.

Bicycling with Your Baby

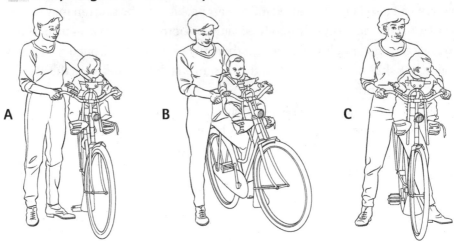

9.15. Bicycling with baby
A. The seat should be so low that your feet can reach the ground.
B. To mount the bike, first lift one foot over the frame.
C. While sitting on the bike, put either foot on the ground before pedaling.

Place your bike to your side. Lift your child with his or her back to you. Hold your knees outward and lift the child against your chest. Stand by the bicycle and put the child into the bicycle seat.

Child Car Seats

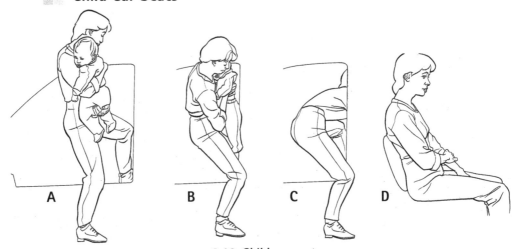

9.16. Child car seats
A. Hold your child against you as you step into the car with one leg.
B. Stabilize your weight through your knees. C. Attach the safety harness quickly.
D. For Mom, a back support cushion can be helpful while driving.

If you have a small car it may not be possible to sit in the backseat while you secure your child in the car seat. If this is the case, here is an easy and pain-free technique. Remember to keep one leg outside the car when you're placing the child in the car seat.

Tips and Reminders

❑ Don't wear shoes that don't have traction.

❑ If you like to sleep with a cushion between your legs, use a Velcro band to attach the cushion to your thigh.

❑ Avoid activities that exercise the muscles on the inside of your upper thighs (adductors).

❑ When preparing to go cycling, try your bicycle seat in different positions and see which is the most comfortable. Be aware that specially designed seats are available for women.

❑ If you're not strong enough to pedal a bike, consider using an electric bike.

❑ If possible, don't take your children with you when you go shopping.

❑ When you are buying a stroller, make sure that the handle is long enough to allow you to bend your arms when you push it and that the stroller is easy to steer.

❑ Choose a changing table that is high enough so you will not have to bend over. Your elbows should be at a ninety-degree angle when you change the baby's diaper.

❑ Choose a crib with a base that can be adjusted for height.

❑ Don't carry a car seat with a child in it. Take your child out and carry him or her separately. It's better to make an extra trip.

❑ Let someone else vacuum; instead, use a broom with a long-handled dustpan. This is also a good way to pick up small toys.

❑ Big boxes are a good place to store toys, especially if the boxes have wheels.

❑ Don't pick up after your kids all day long. Give the kids a place (such as a rug) where they can leave their toys. You can keep the rest of the house the way you want it.

❏ If the kitchen counter is too low, elevate your work surface so you can work at a more comfortable level. For example, you can create a raised counter area by placing a cutting board on top of an overturned dish basin.

❏ If you have a mail slot through which mail drops onto the floor, hang a tray or basket beneath it to catch the mail.

❏ Running after children is something you can only attempt after your pelvis is strong again. If you want to take your toddler for a walk, consider using a harness to attach the child to the stroller.

❏ Give your children the room and the time to become people in their own right. Don't do everything for them. They have to learn some things for themselves, and it's not so terrible if they don't yet do tasks as well as you do.

❏ Hurrying around is rarely a good idea.

❏ Every now and then do something special for yourself. If you are happy, your children will be happy. Give yourself some quality time.

PART IV

Pregnancy and Beyond

Labor and Delivery

What Happens Next? Following Up on Patient Stories

10

Labor and Delivery

Ronnie had three treatments during her first pregnancy. Following her therapy she practiced yoga. In the following note she describes her delivery and recovery period:

> *The midwife quickly pushed my legs up and pressed my abdomen to speed up delivery. Scarce attention was paid to the problems I'd had with pelvic instability. For twenty-four hours I practiced the right sitting and lying positions and did some exercises, and the pain diminished. A week later I no longer had problems.*

In earlier chapters I described the difference certain exercises made in my quality of life during my third pregnancy. I was able to keep walking right until my delivery. On the day I was due, I comfortably walked through the woods, washed windows, and had my baby at home.

My third child was large. As happened with the first two, this baby got stuck at the shoulders. For the first time, I could feel how the sacral bone tilts forward and the hipbones move into the correct position to allow the baby enough room to be born. It took ten hours for my third child to be delivered, but the duration of the labor did not seem important in light of how proud I felt of my body.

I'll never forget the recovery period after the third birth. Once the stitches were in place, I could stand up to take a shower, and a few hours later I could tense my stomach muscles. I could put my legs in the air and make bicycling movements as I lay on my back. And I could sleep on my stomach for the first time since my car accident ten years earlier.

Preparing for Delivery

Over the past decade, my colleagues and I have followed many women who suffered from pregnancy-related pelvic dysfunction. The use of forceps, vacuum extraction (ventouse), Caesarean section, or stimulating medication didn't have any effect on overall recovery. Ninety percent of the women we observed had a successful recovery; eighteen months after delivery, on average, they showed no symptoms of pelvic or back pain.

Only two factors related to delivery appeared to be significantly associated with recovery from pelvic pain:

1. Those women who experienced extreme, unbearable pain during their delivery were more at risk for a slow recovery. Thirty-seven percent of the symptomatic women in our study had experienced extreme pain, compared to 13 percent of the asymptomatic women.

2. The longer the duration of the delivery, counted from the first subjective sign—contraction or losing fluid—the greater the risk of slow recovery. Thirty-five percent of the symptomatic women delivered after more than eighteen hours, compared to 14 percent of the asymptomatic women.

Be aware that you can reduce your chance of a very long or extremely painful delivery if you exercise on a regular basis. The exercises described in this book help to correct any misalignment of the pelvis and help to keep it aligned so that the delivery can proceed without complications. In addition, learn how to relax and try to think positive thoughts. Remind yourself that your prognosis is good and that correction of your pelvis is always possible, even when your baby has just been born.

Once your labor has begun, breathe quietly into your stomach (the same breathing pattern one learns in childbirth classes). Cope with the contractions in a way that feels comfortable for you—lying, sitting, or leaning forward with your head on your hands. Try to keep walking if you can and if your health-care professional says it's okay. You can also do a "contraction dance," either together with your partner or by yourself (see Figure 10.1 on the next page). Practice it regularly before delivery.

Contraction Dance

☐ Stand on both legs and lift your stomach with your hands. Keep your shoulders low and lift from your elbows.

☐ Have your partner stand behind you, pressed against you, also holding your stomach with his hands.

☐ Standing in that position, gracefully sway in unison, first to one side and then the other.

☐ Together bend the left knee, and with a gliding motion let your weight sink onto that knee.

☐ Now gradually, rhythmically, move back to the middle, and then sink onto the right knee.

☐ Continue, slowly alternating the movement. You can repeat these movements quietly and with great concentration for as long as you desire.

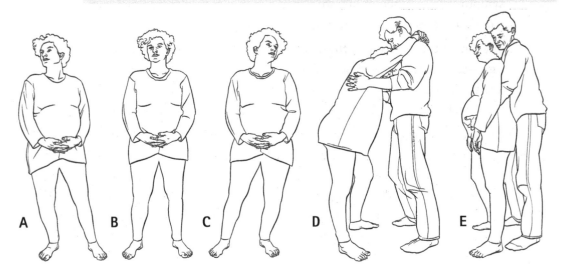

10.1. Contraction dance
A, B, and C. Pull your stomach up with your hands, and move
rhythmically back and forth, keeping your knee bent above the foot.
D and E. Perform these graceful movements in tandem with your partner.

The contraction dance really helps to balance your pelvis and prepare it for delivery. The movements allow gravity to advance your labor and make it easier for your baby to push against the cervix, opening it. By moving rhythmically, you relax your pelvic-floor muscles, which is necessary for the baby's easy passage.

During Labor

During labor it's important to maintain pelvic balance. You can accomplish this by assuming a comfortable, supported position. Try the following:

☐ Lie on your back with your legs bent, knees turned outward, and the soles of your feet on the bed (see Figure 10.2A).

☐ Lie on your back holding your legs up (see Figure 10.2B).

☐ Sit on a barstool, feet resting on the floor, with your weight distributed evenly between both legs (see Figure 10.2C).

Many of my patients have used the position illustrated in Figure 10.2B and have found it very helpful.

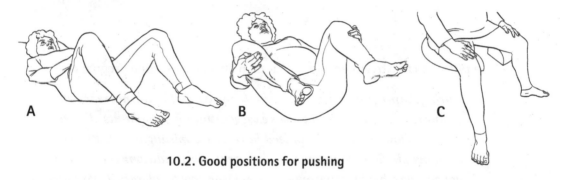

10.2. Good positions for pushing

Some women hear a crackling sound around the symphysis pubis during labor, which happens when the symphysis has created a vacuum. This is nothing to worry about; it will not cause further pelvic complaints. Pelvic complaints happen when the pelvis is not realigned after delivery.

Don't be afraid of labor. If you need to, right after delivery you will be able to adjust your pelvis with a few balancing exercises while you're still mildly sedated. In the first few months after delivery, the joints are still very flexible, so whatever is crooked can be set right.

Once you have delivered your baby, you can use an abdominal dressing or wear underpants that include a snug support panel to hold the sacrum in place. If the delivery doesn't go as well as you'd hoped, know that you can still correct any resulting misalignment, even years later. Just as you learned to function with a changed pelvis, you can learn to restore the correct function.

11

What Happens Next?
Following Up on Patient Stories

Jennifer had two treatments for pelvic pain during her second pregnancy:

During the pregnancy there was definitely pelvic pain. I did not react when people told me they thought I was exaggerating my complaints; diagnostic tests showed that I did indeed have pelvic misalignment. I learned from my physiotherapist how to "self-treat" the condition. The pain did not go away, but by doing my exercises I was able to tolerate it. My home delivery was problem-free. Until the baby's head crowned, I was able to lie on my side. I was very happy that I had no symptoms following the delivery. After three hours, I could climb the stairs and had no problems sitting in a chair. My posture is also good and I can walk without wobbling.

Tina, whom you first met in Chapters 4 and 5 and who underwent four treatments during pregnancy, wrote to me two months after her delivery:

I am able to walk fast again with my older son running after me, whereas before he would run ahead of me. This has to do with strength, and I have achieved it with exercise. I no longer have any pain.

Throughout this book you have read excerpts from letters that were sent to me by women whom I treated when I first began working with pelvic pain patients, in the few months after I delivered my third child. This chapter follows up on the progress of many of these patients.

Women Who Received Treatment During Pregnancy

How did women fare who received two to five treatments during pregnancy?

Sophie (Chapters 4 and 9) wrote that at thirty-eight weeks of gestation she could only walk for about fifteen minutes but had no problem sitting or lying down. Doing chores and caring for her children were going well. Walking up the stairs, riding a bike, and grocery shopping were also going reasonably well.

Following delivery she had no problems for three weeks. Then she started to experience some discomfort again. Two weeks later the pain diminished somewhat. Spreading her legs apart was still not easy, but she could do everything else. Five weeks after delivery she told me that she doubted if she would ask for another treatment, and she thought the pain was diminishing.

For *Ronnie* (Chapters 4 and 9), after thirty-eight weeks of pregnancy everything was going quite well. Lying down, taking care of chores, and making love were reasonably pain free. A week after delivery she found she was too tired to take a long walk. Although she had not yet attempted to ride a bike, play sports, make love, or go shopping, everything else was quite positive.

During the delivery, she experienced a lot of pain in her pelvis. Right after she received stitches, however, she did a symmetry exercise that properly aligned her pelvis. A week later I received an enthusiastic phone call from her telling me that her baby was doing quite nicely.

Miranda (Chapter 5) was able to do all activities well and without restriction two months after delivery. She wrote that her lower-back pain sometimes returned during her period. Two weeks after delivery it seemed as if the pain was coming back, but fortunately, continuing to perform her exercises eliminated the problem.

Four months after delivery, *Adrienne* (Chapter 6) could walk or bike for two and a half hours, walk up the stairs, sit, and lie down without any problem. Doing chores, taking care of her child, going shopping, and making love were all going reasonably well. At that point she wanted to play sports again, so she came in for a session to learn a few more exercises. The pain went away after the first treatment, during which she could once again lie down with her legs held symmetrically apart. (Exercises performed while sitting in the tailor's position, such as those illustrated in Figures 6.1, 6.2, and 6.4, are important to make the back supple and strong again.)

Six months after the birth of her child, *Joanna* (Chapters 5 and 7) reported that her ability to sit comfortably was much improved. This is important to her, since her job involves long periods of sitting and the chair she uses at work isn't well designed. All other movements were also going well.

Janice (Chapter 3) reported that six months after delivery she was able to perform all activities reasonably or very well, with the exception of playing sports. Janice also referred her mother to me for treatment. Janice's mother had suffered from the same problem in her lower back for years. (Her mother is also a physiotherapist.) After a week Janice sent me a note: "My mother called from her vacation. She was walking in the mountains. Every now and then she would try her newest exercise, the tailor's position. She's very happy because before the treatment she couldn't get into that position."

For *Karen* (Chapters 5 and 7), everything was continuing to go well when she checked in seven months after the delivery. She reported having some symptoms when lying in bed. Sometimes she was having problems lifting her child from a squatting position, but no other complaints.

Women Who Received Treatment after Delivery

What happened to the women who received two to ten treatments following their delivery?

Francine (Chapter 2) had three treatments after delivery. Three months later, she had no problem taking twenty-minute walks. She also reported that other types of activity presented no problem, regardless of how long she engaged in them.

Michelle (Chapter 4) had five treatments starting six weeks after delivery. After six months she wrote that she no longer had any pain. She could carry out all of her daily activities without restriction. However, she was not yet seriously playing sports. On one occasion she ran for about ten minutes and felt some pain, but afterward she had no complaints.

Janet (Chapter 1), who had nine treatments in the space of four months and who wrote to me when her daughter was a year old, said that climbing stairs, lying down, riding a bike, and cleaning the house were going well. However, shopping and playing sports were not yet pain-free. In every other area she was doing reasonably well. The longest she could walk, sit up, or ride a bike was for half an hour. However, she could recline with a cushion under her knees for two hours. She reported doing the exercises every day and felt that she was continuing to improve. A month later I spoke to her again; she had begun working with a personal trainer on the goal of strengthening her abdominal muscles and had taken up her old hobby of deep-sea diving. She said she experienced much less pelvic pain. However, although it had lessened, she still had persistent back pain. Over the next couple of months she came to my office a few times for treatment.

Ellen (Chapter 2), who was treated three times, had no more problems when we corresponded seventeen months after she delivered her third baby.

Yvonne (Chapter 1), who has two children, was still walking with crutches when she first came to see me. She underwent four treatments. After the first treatment she no longer needed to use crutches or a pelvic sling. She can now walk for about an hour at a time. Riding a bike and playing sports are still somewhat uncomfortable, but all other activities are progressing. She has the potential for additional improvement if she continues to follow the program. She writes, "My normal life is going reasonably well, and that was not the case before these treatments. There is a definite improvement when it comes to the pain. The symptoms do recur, but I no longer get up in pain every morning."

Pauline (Chapter 7) had five treatments, starting a year after her delivery. Her child is now almost two years old. She was treated for the last time about nine months ago. She reports that everything has been going well, including resting, making love, and playing sports.

Ingrid (Chapter 5) underwent seven treatments. She had endured complaints since her first delivery. Fifteen months after the birth of her third child, and following the treatments and the program of exercises, she reported that lying down, sitting, shopping, and all other daily activities were going reasonably well. The only thing she had not yet resumed was playing sports. She no longer has any pain.

Jackie (Chapter 4) had ten treatments over a three-month period when her daughter was four years old. She recently reported that her daily activities were going reasonably well and that she could walk and ride a bike for hours. She also said that she occasionally has complaints when she has her period or if she pulls a muscle or sustains an injury. She once again plays sports and doesn't feel the need to return for treatment. She has regained control over her body.

The cases described thus far in the book were collected in the Netherlands almost a decade ago. I have heard similar cases over and over again in the past ten years, told by women of many different races from all over the world. At first, scientists thought that pelvic instability was a Northern European problem, but nowadays we know that pregnancy-related pelvic pain is experienced by women around the globe. We have been able to answer many questions about possible causes for this condition, and the search continues. By reading Parts I through IV of this book you have become fully informed about the signs and symptoms of pregnancy-related pelvic pain. You have studied the exercises and postures that will give you control over your pelvis and lower back. If you are interested in scientific research, read Part V.

PART V

Scientific Research and Clinical Information for Therapists

CECILE RÖST graduated in 1985 as a physiotherapist from the Academie voor Fysiotherapie Jan van Essen, in Amsterdam, Netherlands, and as an Orthopedic Manual Therapist in 2004. She has also received the following training:

- Pregnancy Education (Amsterdam). This course qualified her to teach pregnancy gymnastics. For seven years she has taught yoga, gymnastics, and baby massage to pregnant women

- Orthopedic Healing for Physiotherapists (Delft, Netherlands)

- Sensory Integration (Haarlem, Netherlands)

- Neurological Development Methods (Antwerp and Gits, Belgium)

She also presents workshops and lectures to train fitness trainers, nurses, midwives, physiotherapists, and doctors on the use of her method of therapy. Her first scientific study of these treatment methods was published in *Spine* in 2004. Her next study was published in 2006 in *Acta Obstetricia et Gynecologica Scandinavica*.

12

Analysis of Research Findings

As described earlier in the book, I initially became interested in possible treatments for pregnancy-related pelvic pain as a patient. During my third pregnancy, I was teaching yoga and discovered that I could reduce my pelvic pain by following specific exercises. I taught myself to once again walk and move comfortably. Since then, thousands of women with pelvic pain have been referred to me by doctors, other therapists, midwives, or pelvic pain patients. Over time I began to see patterns in the histories described by these patients. Numerous conversations with doctors, scientists, midwives, and therapists followed.

Curious about the circumstances of these patients, I created a list of questions and began collecting data. I hoped to get answers to such questions as the following:

- Is there a difference between the onset of pelvic pain in women who have a job outside the home and women who don't work outside the home?
- When did the complaints start?
- Are earlier (vague) complaints of the back, hip, knee, and feet any indication for the later development of pelvic pain?
- Is there a relationship between playing sports and pelvic pain?
- Does an earlier physical trauma play a role in the development of pelvic pain?

This chapter analyzes my findings to these and other questions. My analysis is based on medical histories, patient evaluations (particularly of the hip and pelvic area), and review of the latest research. With this information, I formulated a hypothesis regarding the cause(s) of pelvic pain (see Chapters 3 and 13).

As the amount of data I collected piled up over the years, a Dutch foundation for orthopedic research, Het Annafonds, partially financed two epidemiologic studies. The Department of General Practice at the Erasmus University Rotterdam was willing to assist and guide me and my colleague, Drs. Jacqueline Kaiser, in this huge project. In November 2004 the first study was published in the journal *Spine* (Röst et al. 2004). In 2006 a second study was published in *Acta Obstetricia et Gynecologica Scandinavica* (Röst et al. 2006). Some results from these studies are mentioned in this book. None of the results contradict the conclusions I drew from my first pilot study, which is described in this chapter. In addition, a North-American review concerning backaches related to pregnancy was conducted in 2003 by S.M. Wang. The abstract of the review remarks: Gestational backache is a substantial problem and can have a significant impact on a pregnant woman's daily activities. Nonpharmacological/complementary treatments such as posture adjustment, acupuncture, physical therapy, physiotherapy, yoga, and chiropractic may become the first line of treatment options. In labor backache the posture of the parturient can have an effect in decreasing the intensity of pain. Allopathic medicine, regional techniques (epidural), and complementary interventions are routinely given to parturients. However, there is a major perception of differences among midwives, obstetricians, and anesthesiologists in terms of the risks and benefits of labor epidural analgesia. Postpartum backache is usually self-limited, but for some mothers the pain can last from a few months to several years. Early literature suggested that this problem was associated with the use of epidurals, but recent data in the literature deny such an association. Since the 1990s numerous studies have been published concerning peripartum pelvic pain, pregnancy-related pelvic pain, pelvic instability, reliability of sacroiliac tests, form and force closure of the sacroiliac joints, and muscular stability systems of the pelvis and lower back. Researchers are now studying the contribution of emotional and psychological factors to chronic pelvic pain. It is astonishing to observe how study results validate the treatment approach that is described in this book.

Terminology

Orthopedic problems associated with delivery are often lumped into the general category of pelvic instability. Typical features of pregnancy-related pelvic pain include sciatic conditions during pregnancy, lower-back pain, sacral pain, symptoms of trochanteric bursitis, and gapping or slipping of the pubic bones at the symphysis pubis (symphysiolysis). As I touched on in Chapter 1, whether "pelvic instability" is the correct term for pregnancy-related pelvic pain remains open to discussion. Are the complaints caused by hypermobility in one or both sacroiliac (SI) joints? And even so, couldn't a stiff SI joint be the cause of too much freedom of movement in the other SI joint? In the United States the terms "SI joint dysfunction" (SIJD) and "sacroiliac subluxation" are commonly used to describe a stiff or displaced joint. Furthermore, isn't there always some degree of joint and ligament instability present during pregnancy? In my opinion pelvic hypermobility is not a pathologic condition during pregnancy or in the first months postpartum. The pelvis should be more mobile to allow for childbirth. Complaints arise when for one reason or another the woman is not in control of her pelvic joints.

In this part of the book, I would prefer to speak of pregnancy-related pelvic pain (PRP) and save the term "pelvic instability" for patients who are diagnosed with this condition by doctors and who still have problems with daily activities after the first few months of motherhood.

Methodology

As of June 2006, my colleagues and I had treated approximately three thousand women with pelvic complaints, of whom two thousand were pregnant. The most consistent positive finding in pregnancy was Patrick's Sign, in which painful symptoms are reproduced when the hip is externally rotated. In 77 percent of the studied women a positive finding such as pain or different endfeel was present. Sixty-six percent of the patients reported difficulty when given the active straight-leg raising test.

The results of the very first 140 women we treated became the basis for Pilot Study A; the background details of 130 women comprise Pilot Study B (see below). The women in our pilot studies varied in age from twenty to forty-two years. Their nationalities included Dutch, Turkish, Surinamese, Moroccan, and Egyptian. (The results of the two pilot studies formed the basis for a later epidemiologic study, published in 2004, of 870 pregnant women; Röst et al. 2004.)

Pilot Study A (Sample Size: n = 140)

Working Outside the Home vs. Stay-at-Home Moms

Approximately half of the patients worked at jobs that often required heavy lifting, a great deal of standing, or physical caregiving. Nurses and other hospital workers made up the majority of this sample, with therapists and teachers also well represented. In summary:

- ❑ 51 percent (n = 72) worked at jobs that often required heavy lifting.
- ❑ 38 percent (n = 53) had sedentary jobs.
- ❑ 11 percent (n = 15) did not work outside the home.

Compare these percentages, graphically illustrated in Figure 12.2, with the percentages of women who hold these types of jobs in the Dutch population in general (see Figure 12.1).

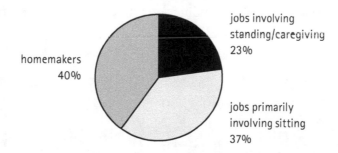

12.1. Division per occupation of women ages 25 to 44 in the Netherlands
(SOURCE: Centraal Bureau Statistieken, "Enquete Beroeps Bevolking" [Official Dutch Statistics from the Profession Questionnaire of 1997])

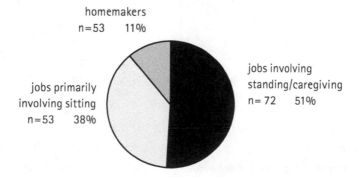

12.2. Division per occupation of women with PRP, ages 20 to 42, in the Netherlands

Conclusions Regarding Occupations

Of the 140 women with pelvic pain whom we studied, the majority worked in a caregiving occupation. Mothers who were full-time homemakers (i.e., who did not work outside the home) were in the minority in this patient population, compared to the number of women with a job.

Those women who work outside the home can be further divided into three groups: women whose jobs entail standing/lifting, women whose jobs primarily involve sitting, and women whose jobs primarily involve doing housework.

When Complaints First Occur

The initial complaints began during the first pregnancy in the majority of all three groups (respectively 63 percent, 58 percent, 60 percent). The women with sedentary jobs and those who were full-time homemakers often did not come in for therapy during their first pregnancy. In comparison, the women with jobs that entailed a great deal of standing and lifting were more likely to seek treatment.

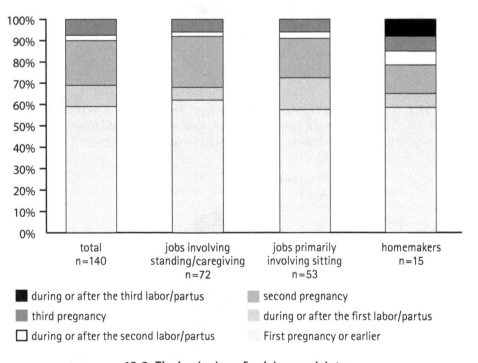

12.3. The beginning of pelvic complaints

Conclusion Regarding Timing of First Need for Therapy

More than two-thirds of the patients came for therapy during their second pregnancy.

Earlier Back, Hip, Knee, and Foot Complaints

In the patients surveyed, it seems that 71 percent had previously experienced back pain. These complaints were sometimes vague, occurring only during ovulation, before menstruation, or as the result of lifting something heavy. Hip complaints, such as a "snapping hip," had been experienced by 23 percent of the women, and 29 percent had experienced problems with their feet, ranging from fractures to sprains to overpronation. Almost half (46 percent) of the women had problems with their knees, in almost all cases, unilateral chondromalacia patella.

Only 11 percent had never had any problems with their back or legs. Only 8 percent (11 patients) had never experienced knee, hip, or foot problems.

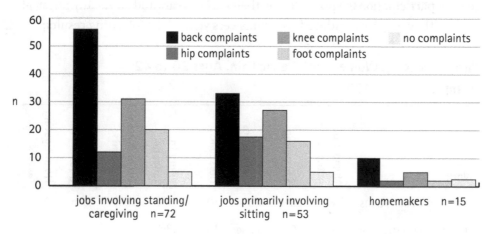

12.4. Complaints that presented before pelvic pain began

Conclusions Regarding Earlier Complaints

❑ In all three groups, the most common earlier complaint was low back pain, followed by knee problems.

❑ Isolated knee, hip, or foot complaints seldom led to PRP.

❑ A combination of earlier experiences with back, knee, hip, and foot problems was common with PRP patients.

Pilot Study B (Sample Size: n = 130)

Sports, Physical Trauma, and PRP

After speaking with literally dozens of patients, I began to notice that certain sports seemed to be mentioned more often than others—especially swimming, gymnastics, and horseback riding. In these activities one closes the legs with a forceful motion and there is a tendency toward muscular imbalance: overdevelopment of the muscles of the pelvic floor and inner thigh and relative underuse of the external rotator muscles and thigh abductors. Having been very active in any of these three sports in youth appeared to be significantly related to the seriousness of complaints in pregnancy, as shown in the second published study. Multivariate analysis shows swimming to be the activity most strongly related to PRP. (This topic was touched on earlier in the book.)

Another common occurrence is an injury to the tailbone, either from a fall or as the result of a car accident, that appeared to cause no further serious consequences at the time of injury. I began routinely asking my patients about any intensive participation in sports during their earlier years and about any physical trauma they may have endured. Their answers yielded the following results:

Patient History, Women with Pelvic Pain, Ages 20 to 42
(sample size: n = 130)

Work	Number of patients	Swimming	Gymnastics	Horseback riding	Injury to tailbone	Other types of accidents	General trauma	No mitigating factors
Standing occupations	62	29%	26%	10%	5%	18%	6%	31%
Sitting occupations	48	29%	29%	10%	33%	19%	8%	6%
Homemaking	20	40%	10%	20%	35%	15%	10%	3%
Totals	130	31%	25%	12%	20%	18%	8%	19%

The above information was compared with that of a control group (n = 100) of women who did not have pelvic complaints either during or after their pregnancy and who had small children at the time of the study. The control group consisted of a matched sampling of women approached at shopping centers, at sports programs, and in various neighborhoods. The ages were similar, as were other demographic factors.

Incidence of Pelvic Pain, by Occupation

Distribution	n	%
Standing/lifting/caregiving	62	48
Sedentary	48	37
Stay-at-home mom	20	15
Total	130	100

Personal History, Women with and Without Pelvic Pain, Ages 20 to 42

	Number of Respondents	Swimming	Gymnastics	Horseback riding	Injury to tailbone	Other types of accidents	General trauma	No mitigating factors
No PRP	100	18%	14%	6%	9%	10%	4%	58%
PRP	130	31%	25%	12%	20%	18%	8%	19%

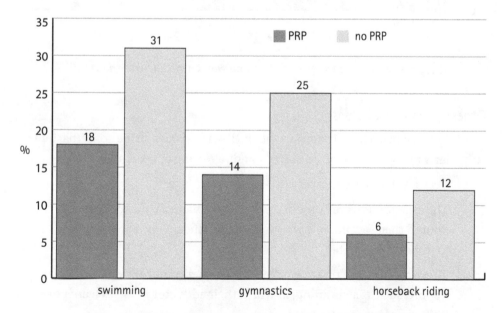

12.5. Intensive participation in certain sports during youth
among women with and without PRP

Conclusions Regarding PRP and a Background in Specific Sports

A third of the patients swam on a regular basis, a fourth took part in gymnastics, and about 12 percent rode horses. These are all larger percentages than those found in the control group. Individuals who experienced PRP were nearly twice as likely to have participated in these sports. These are all activities that tend to overdevelop muscles in the inner thigh, possibly predisposing one to pelvic instability. Research into other sports did not prove of interest.

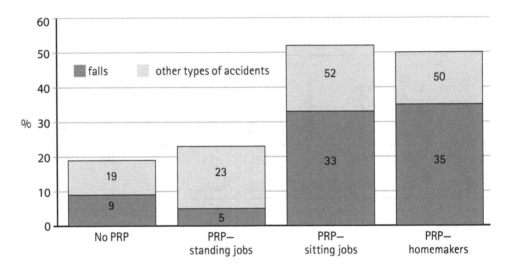

12.6. Earlier trauma experienced among women with and without PRP

Other General Conclusions

❑ The vast majority of the group with PRP worked outside the home, particularly in jobs that involved either standing/lifting or sedentary work.

❑ Very few PRP patients were full-time homemakers.

❑ The exceptions were homemakers who had had a car accident or a fall that injured their sacrum in a way that was significant enough for them to remember it years later.

❑ These trends were true regardless of whether or not they participated in a sport, such as swimming, in which their adductor muscles were potentially overdeveloped.

❑ Among the women without PRP, 58 percent did not have predisposing factors.

❑ The percentage of women having experienced earlier traumas was noticeably higher in women with PRP who had a sedentary job or were full-time homemakers.

❑ Trauma did not seem to be a factor for women with PRP who worked in a profession involving a great deal of standing, lifting, or physically caring for patients. These women experienced physical trauma with the same frequency as members of the control group.

❑ Among homemakers and sedentary workers with PRP, a history of participation in sports that overexercise the adductor muscles did not seem to be a factor.

❑ There were almost no women with PRP who did not have a job outside the home.

13

Risk Factors

Pelvic pain during pregnancy is common, with incidence rates worldwide of 48 to 56 percent. In 2007 an American study of 599 low-socioeconomic pregnant women was published (Skaggs et al. 2007) that showed even higher numbers within this particular population:

> *Women completed an author-generated musculoskeletal survey in the second trimester of their pregnancy that addressed pain history, duration, location, and intensity, as well as activities of daily living, treatment frequency, and satisfaction with treatment. Sixty-seven percent of the total population reported musculoskeletal pain, and nearly half presented with a multi-focal pattern of pain that involved 2 or more sites. Twenty-one percent reported severe pain intensity rated on a numerical rating scale. Eighty percent of women experiencing pain slept less than 4 hours per night and 75% of these women took pain medications. Importantly, 85% of the women surveyed perceived that they had not been offered treatment for their musculoskeletal disorders.*

Although a large number of possible risk factors have been studied, the exact cause of pelvic pain during pregnancy remains unclear. Taking a closer look at some study results can help us understand the phenomenon of PRP.

Pregnancy

In general, it can be said that strong pelvic pain is directly related to pregnancy. About 45 percent of all pregnant women and 25 percent of all women postpartum suffer from pregnancy-related pelvic and/or low back pain. During pregnancy, serious pain occurs in about 25 percent of patients and severe disability in about 8 percent. After pregnancy, problems are serious in about 7 percent of women (Wu et al. 2004, Pregnancy-related pelvic girdle pain). In 60 percent of PRP patients, the pain is noticeable during the first pregnancy; 37 percent of patients have pain eighteen months after delivery (Ostgaard and Anderson 1992). In comparison, 10 percent of the patients treated during pregnancy by the method described in this book had symptoms of pain and experienced at least one difficulty in daily activities, on average eighteen months postpartum (Röst et al. 2006).

Pregnancy is also a risk factor in the development of *chronic* low back pain (Mens et al. 1996). Frequent lifting and standing, combined with caring for children or patients, increases the chance of pelvic pain during pregnancy or delivery (Ostgaard et al. 1993; Mens 1995; and my own research, Chapter 12 of this book). Other factors during gestation that play a role in the development of pelvic pain include muscle imbalance, the weight of the fetus, carrying twins, and gaining weight rapidly, which can weaken stomach muscles (Ostgaard et al. 1993; Mens 1995; Mens et al. 1996). In my research no evidence was found that any of these factors influenced the prognosis (Röst et al. 2006).

Greater mobility of the pelvis is seen in all pregnant women. Many authors surmise that this loosening of the ligaments is caused by the hormone relaxin (MacLennan 1991), which has been associated with pelvic pain during pregnancy (Mens et al. 1996; Engelen et al. 1995). According to Bjorklund et al. (1999, Sonographic assessment of symphyseal joint distention), however, there is no evidence that the degree of symphyseal distension determines the severity of pelvic pain during pregnancy or after childbirth. However, another study reveals that the majority of pregnant women with a symphyseal width of more than 9.5 millimeters experience symphyseal pain (Schoellner et al. 2001). Women with PRP have positive provocative tests and ligament and muscular tenderness. Bad coping strategies may be an explanation for why these women develop complaints, according to Hansen et al. (2005). Recent research indicates a significant relationship between the development of complaints and psychological factors (e.g., the woman experiences a heavy workload due to either her own or a colleague's pregnancy), former neck injury, fatigue or nausea in the first months of pregnancy, and the knowledge of a history of pregnancy-related pelvic pain in a mother or sister (Röst et al., to be published).

Measurement of sacroiliac joint stiffness with Doppler imaging of vibrations showed that asymmetric laxity of the sacroiliac joints could be related to low-back pain and pelvic pain during and after pregnancy. In PRP patients, a larger difference in mobility of the SI joints is found (Damen et al. 2002). Asymmetry could be the result of a trauma such as falling on one buttock or the tailbone, a car accident, or simply using incorrect postures during pregnancy (e.g., passive weight bearing on one overextended leg).

Injuries and Other Orthopedic Conditions

Earlier experiences of back pain also seem to heighten the risk of PRP (Mens 1995). The combination of earlier back pain and orthopedic problems in the legs, such as chondromalacia patellae or a "snapping hip," seems to occur frequently in PRP patients. Almost half the patients surveyed said they once had a problem with chondromalacia patellae (pilot research, see Figure 12.4 on page 93).

This leads me to believe that a posture with locked knees and a forward-placed pelvis, combined with heavy work, including forward bending or frequent lifting during pregnancy, can cause PRP symptoms. In particular, tasks that require forward tilting of the upper trunk need special attention during and after pregnancy; activation of stabilizing systems is required. Also, women who are in distress about their jobs, or who have responded to hormonal changes with nausea or fatigue, are more at risk of pelvic pain. In my opinion, inattention to the physical changes caused by pregnancy, often in combination with inadequate motor patterns or bad posture, is the main cause of PRP.

Joint Compression: Stability

Normally, only a few degrees of motion are possible in the SI joints. Movement is restricted by the position and form of the joints and by a muscular system that is able to tense the fascia thoracolumbalis. In the self-bracing SI joint compression model (Lee 1996; Don Tigny 1995; Snijders et al. 1995; Vleeming et al. 1992), the nutation (forward nodding movement or anterior tilt) of the sacrum plays an important role in stabilization of the pelvis and lower back. Sacral nutation is a close-pack position that occurs upon lumbopelvic loading. It is thought to be the most stable position for the SI joint, and it is controlled by muscular and ligamentous attachments. This happens when the pelvic ilia cantilever relatively backward. Sacral nutation is needed to help stabilize the pelvis enough to be able to lift things (Don Tigny 1995). The self-bracing model implies that the pelvis is most stable when the back is in a normal lordotic curve and the pelvis is rotated slightly backward, as occurs when you bend your knees slightly while standing.

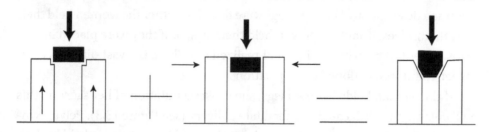

13.1. Joint compression model (Source: Vleeming et al. 1995)

During pregnancy the form-closure model (see Figures 13.1 and 13.2A) is slightly disturbed by the ligamental laxity of the SI joints; extra force closure is needed. Many SI-related complaints during pregnancy are provoked by forward tilting of the trunk. If the stabilizing muscles do not provide enough support, the self-bracing mechanism will no longer work as efficiently and the sacrum will begin to "hang" or glide unilaterally toward the stomach, causing sacroiliac subluxation (see Figure 13.2B). The sacrum rotates on a longitudinal/oblique axis if there is a difference in laxity between the two SI joints, causing pain in the lower back or somewhere in or around the pelvis. Form and force closure are both important in preventing the sacrum from gliding into an unnatural position, thus disturbing the normal alignment of the pelvis.

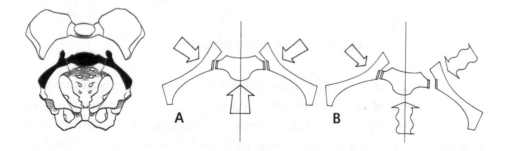

13.2. Horizontal view of the SI joints
A. Normal alignment
B. One-sided hypermobile SI joint due to weakened muscles
(here the ilium is shifted forward)

Delivery

A flexed position of the legs during birth has been described as a possible cause of PRP (Mens et al. 1996). The research does not include further distinctions, such as a description of how the legs were flexed, whether the women held their legs themselves, if another person held their legs, or if they were placed in stir-rups. After talking with a midwife, I realized that there is a vast difference between the aforementioned three positions.

If the woman holds her own legs, she causes a nutation of her sacrum; this will enlarge the birth canal and facilitate delivery (see Figure 13.3). Pelvic symmetry is likely to remain intact. If her legs are placed in supports or held back by another person while the woman pushes during delivery, she may react by pushing her legs down and away from her. Doing this causes a counternutation shift and the birth canal narrows. In this case, delivery will be hindered. Further, in the case of two helpers, each helper may use different amounts of strength to hold his or her assigned leg, which may twist the pelvis.

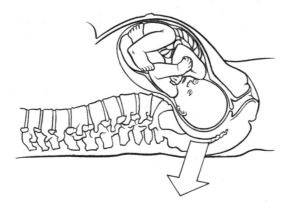

13.3. Nutation expands the birth canal.

For most women, delivery is uncomplicated and does not result in pelvic pain (Engelen et al. 1995). A rupture of the pubic symphysis takes place in as few as one in twenty-two hundred deliveries and heals quickly. When the pubic symphysis heals properly, there is no increased risk of a Caesarean section during a future pregnancy (Schwartz et al. 1985). (One disadvantage of a C-section is that the procedure involves severing abdominal muscles. This slows the healing and strengthening of these stabilizing muscles; as a result, the excessive motion of the sacrum may be a problem for a longer period of time.)

Prognosis for PRP patients is independent of the type of delivery (Röst et al. 2006). Long duration of the partus and experience of extreme pain during delivery were the only significant factors we found to have a negative effect on the prognosis. Earlier studies found that chronic pelvic pain lasted, on average, over six years (Brynhildsen et al. 1998). However, overall prognosis of the patients who were treated as described in this book during pregnancy was very good.

Asymmetry in the Pelvis

Pelvic asymmetry is often noticeable in PRP patients. In general, one ilium is rotated forward in comparison to the other ilium. Radiating pain is usually felt on one side—in one buttock, thigh, hip, or groin.

With an X ray you can see how, when a PRP patient stands on one leg, both pubic bones may twist toward each other. When she stands on the other leg the same twist does not occur (Engelen et al. 1995). Standard X-ray research can show the initial stages of symphysiolysis, but over a longer period of time there is often a normal distance between the two halves of the pubic bones, typically three to five millimeters (Van Vugt 1998).

Note that when pain is experienced in the pubic symphysis, difficulty in using one leg usually exists. PRP patients tend to prefer standing on one leg and seem to favor the side with the SI pain. By testing the force of the hip and leg muscles against resistance (using the standard manual muscle test), you can see a clear difference between the degree of pain experienced in the two legs.

The active straight-leg raising (ASLR) test (Mens 1996; Van Vugt 1998; see page 114) often shows a difference in sensation between the two legs. Also, in the case of PRP, you can almost always see a clear difference in the height of the knees when the person is lying down and spreading her legs with knees and hips bent. When performing this exercise, pain is experienced first in the adductor muscles, but the pain then moves to the back to the sacroiliac region. Symphyseal pain can be caused by muscle guarding; it makes sense that the pain is experienced right where the tensed muscles are attached, at the pubic bone. The noticeable difference in height of the knees is probably caused by asymmetrical tension of the adductor and pelvic-floor muscles. Instability of both SI joints would, in the case of laxity, not likely cause any limitations in the outward movement of the flexed legs, unless the sacroiliac joints are subluxated. If hormonal-induced laxity in the pelvic ligaments is the primary cause of PRP, the often-seen limitation in the mobility of only one leg in the above-mentioned position is difficult to explain because gravitational forces would lower the legs more easily when joints are lax.

However, if one or both SI joints were blocked in an unnatural position, it would explain the painful limitation of movement and hypertonic adductor and pelvic-floor muscles. The best way to illustrate this is with a cross section of the pelvis at the SI joints (see Figure 13.4).

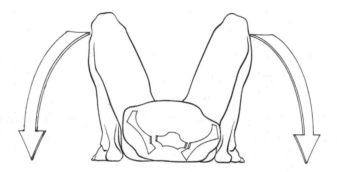

13.4. Sacroiliac subluxation: asymmetrical position of the ilium and sacrum within the torso. The combination of bending the legs and spreading them may be experienced as back pain on the side with the restricted SI joint.

Stability in the Pelvis

This section examines changes that take place in the different parts of the pelvic region during or after pregnancy.

The Sacroiliac Joint (SI Joint)

On each side of the sacrum are the ilia, which are bound to the sacrum through the SI joints. In the front of the pelvis, both ilia are connected at the symphysis pubis, an area of dense fibrous cartilage that can become more pliant during pregnancy to allow the birth canal to enlarge.

Usually, the joint surface of the ilium is slightly convex, and the joint surface of the sacrum is slightly concave. Some people have SI joints in which this concave/convex relationship is reversed, with the ilium concave and the sacrum convex. This allows the ilium to rotate laterally. When there is a disturbance in this activity, it's described as an "inflare" or "outflare" dysfunction of the ilium (see Figure 13.5 ; Greenman 1992). In my practice, flare dysfunctions are often seen in women with PRP, probably caused by pregnancy-related laxity of the SI joint in combination with postural failure. Flare dysfunctions may cause difficulties during labor (see Figure 13.6).

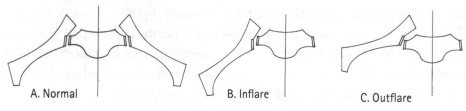

13.5. Inflare and outflare

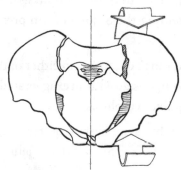

**13.6. The pelvic passageway. In the case of an asymmetry,
the baby may be pushed in the wrong direction during delivery.**

Despite the concave/convex relationship, the SI joints are reasonably flat. Without a compressing force on the joint surface, produced by muscles or mechanical pressure, they cannot handle the vertical shifts or rotations of the ilia that occur in functional movements such as standing up or walking (Snijders et al. 1993). Through small and larger interfaced grooves and ridges in the surface of the joint, and through tension in the ligaments and muscles, a functional balance is achieved between the sacrum and the two ilia. Only a few degrees of motion is possible between the ilium and the sacrum. To function effectively, the surfaces need to push against each other; a certain level of compression, caused by muscle tension or external pressure, is necessary (Ostgaard et al. 1993; Mens 1995; Mens 1996; Lee 1996, Don Tigny 1995; Snijders et al. 1995; Vleeming et al. 1992). To be able to tense the stabilizing muscles of the pelvis and lower back (see Figure 15.1 on page 124), it is necessary that the patient relaxes and controls the adductor muscles and the pelvic-floor muscles (Pool-Goudzwaard et al. 2005). External pressure is increased, for instance, by abducting the legs while seated. All the postures and exercises described in this book are based on these principles of stabilization.

The Pubic Symphysis

The pubic symphysis is the most stable point within the pelvic ring. It rotates back and forth in a sinusoidal curve but moves only slightly to the side (Greenman 1992). To maintain stability in the pelvis, it is not the pubic symphysis that's important (Mens 1995); the sacroiliac joints are the most important structure in providing stability of the pelvis. We need not worry much about the pubic symphysis as a potential cause of pelvic instability as compared to the SI joints.

A number of factors can result in symphyseal pain:

❏ Very early in a pregnancy, the pubic symphysis may swell, which can cause problems by preventing the SI joints from pressing against each other (Mens 1995).

❏ If there is a limited range of motion in either of the SI joints, the other SI joint will have to compensate with an exaggerated movement, resulting in a wringing of the pubic symphysis.

❏ Widening of the pubic symphysis requires exaggerated compensatory movement on the part of the SI joints (see Figures 13.7 and 13.8).

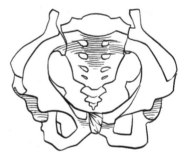

13.7. Mobility for inflare and outflare configurations
HYPERMOBILITY of the symphysis or the blockage of either joint can lead to twisting of the pelvis. This, in turn, can lead to pain and unstable, exaggerated movements of the SI joint, which can slide the ilium into an inflare or outflare position. When this occurs, the position of the hip joint also changes, and the leg turns inward or outward.

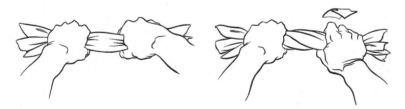

13.8. The pubic symphysis undergoes a wringing action, similar to that involved in wringing out a towel.

The Hip Joints

Over time, chronic PRP patients find that their hip movements are also affected, as if the unstable SI joint were causing the hip joint to assist in maintaining general stability. Conversely, when hips become too stiff, leg movements must recruit the assistance of the SI joints instead of being initiated solely by the hip joints.

Hypothesis: During pregnancy and the months after delivery, the hypermobile ilium can slide along the sacrum, becoming skewed as though it were being twisted. This can happen when the woman flexes, adducts, or endorotates the hip.

If this occurs, the hip joint no longer functions properly—the joint's ability to carry out part of the movement may be curtailed. Women who have had pelvic complaints for an extended period of time after delivery find that they are no longer able to move their legs properly from the hip joints. They lack the coordination required for everyday movements such as walking and turning. Flexion and rotation are no longer fully possible because the ilium and sacrum no longer mesh together properly. Pain in passive testing of flexion and internal rotation of the hip appeared to be related to the seriousness of complaints in pregnant patients (Röst et al. 2004).

Many patients will demonstrate a relative inflare on one side and outflare on the other side of the body. Pain can be located at either SI joint, at the trochanters, or at the pubic symphysis. Some patients only have backache and demonstrate both ilia in the inflare position. To my surprise, in pregnant pelvic pain patients, there appeared to be no differences in test outcome concerning the different pain localizations (Röst et al. 2004). Apparently, tests used to find sacroiliac dysfunction do not add important information during pregnancy.

Inspection of the patient's regular, uncorrected standing posture is the easiest way to start your examination. You may find that one or both femurs are in internal rotation. This happens because the ilium has shifted into an inflare position, placing the hip in an anterior position, and curtailing normal sequences of movement. Palpate the posterior superior iliac spine (PSIS) on both sides and compare the distances to the midline of the sacrum; at the inflare side the distance is largest. In walking, the swing phase no longer begins in the neutral position at the inflare side. From the beginning, there is more external rotation needed for a normal swing phase. It is as if the patient has to search for the correct rotation in both hips before being able to lift a leg from the ground.

Gait in healthy pregnancy is shown to be remarkably normal, but some differences in pelvis-thorax coordination have been detected. In a healthy pregnancy, anti-phase pelvis-thorax coordination, the coordination that is used when someone is walking at higher speed, appears difficult, but less so than in pregnancy-related pelvic pain (Wu et al. 2004, Gait coordination in pregnancy). The anti-phase coordination difficulties can be worked on by a therapist.

The patient has to carry weight on an SI joint in which the bones no longer correctly interface; this may cause extreme pain. The moment when a patient stands on one leg and lifts the other leg is the most painful. It is therefore easier, when walking, to take fewer, bigger steps than to take many smaller steps. Advice traditionally given to pelvic pain patients to be careful, take small steps, and keep the legs together can have immediate negative effects on daily function and can ultimately lead to the loss of hip function. As early as the 1970s, Johnston and Smidt measured hip movements while healthy men were taking part in normal daily activities (1970). From this research it appeared that one needs more than 120 degrees of flex, 20 degrees of abduction, and 20 degrees of external rotation at the hip joints to be able to carry out activities of daily life, such as sitting, getting up, tying shoelaces, crouching, and climbing stairs. In my experience, these numbers are the same for women with pelvic pain. They also need hip mobility to be able to function normally.

14

The First Consultation

A PRP patient's first consultation with a physiotherapist is very important. The physical examination provides valuable information on the extent of symptoms and the degree to which decreased mobility has affected daily functioning. It is essential to rule out other sources of pain and possible coexisting conditions.

The patient may need to be put at ease during the exam and may be afraid to perform normal movements. During the exam, the patient will learn what has been happening to her body, what she can do about it, and why she must perform so many exercises.

Be sure to allow plenty of time for the first exam—at least an hour—so you can take a detailed case history, explain the anatomy and pathology of the pelvis, perform a physical exam, and give the first treatment.

After this session, the patient should come in for half-hour treatments on a weekly basis (or, later, once every two to three weeks) until she is free of symptoms and can function normally.

If the tests are carefully undertaken to the point of pain, the therapist can obtain enough information to treat the patient. When the tests are performed gradually, the pain experienced afterward is quite minimal. In some cases there is no residual pain directly after the exam, in which case the patient can begin doing the symmetry exercise (Chapter 5) immediately. (Clearly the goal is for the patient to be able to do the exercises without pain.)

The following questions and tests can quickly give you a good understanding of the pattern of symptoms. They also provide useful information about the patient's medical background. You can use these tests even if the patient is pregnant. Diagnosis is best made by considering both the symptoms of the patient and the endfeel of the passive tests of the legs. Results of specific tests, such as

ASLR, Patrick's Sign, or resisted adduction, do not add extra information concerning the severity of the complaints, because pain is not always present at the time the tests are administered and the amount of pain may well be influenced by the amount of time the women is required to sit, stand, or lie down immediately prior to the examination (Röst et al. 2004).

Feel free to make photocopies of this chapter so you will have blank charts and questionnaires to use during your exams. For easy printing, this full form is also available for download in an 8½ × 11" format at www.hunterhouse.com.

Case History

Name: _____

Address: _____

City: _____ State: _____ ZIP Code: _____

Telephone: _____

Birth Date: _____

Occupation: _____

Referring physician: _____

Insurance: _____

Ob/Gyn: _____

Midwife: _____

How many weeks pregnant? _____

How many weeks/months/years after delivery? _____

Status

Chief complaint at this point in time: _____

_____

_____

The patient...   _____ wobbles/hobbles/walks with crutches/drags one leg.

_____ is/is not wearing a pelvic sling.

_____ is/is not wearing abdominal support.

_____ does/does not use a wheelchair.

_____ can climb stairs/can climb stairs only with great difficulty/
cannot climb stairs.

Without pain, the patient can: walk for _____ minutes

stand for _____ minutes

lie down for _____ minutes

sit for _____ minutes

ride a bike for _____ minutes

drive a car for _____ minutes

The patient...   _____ sleeps well/reasonably well/badly.

_____ can change positions normally/with difficulty/with pain.

_____ can make love normally/with difficulty/with pain.

Other complaints: _____

_____

_____

_____

General health: _____

_____

_____

_____

Special considerations: _____

_____

_____

_____

Medical History

	First pregnancy	Second pregnancy	Third pregnancy	Fourth pregnancy
Miscarriage/abortion				
Pelvic pain/back pain				
Difficulty walking				
Difficulty changing positions				
Problems with standing and sitting				

	First delivery	Second delivery	Third delivery	Fourth delivery
Date				
Duration of labor				
Forceps or vacuum extraction				
Bleeding				
Extreme pelvic pain				
Recovery				
APGAR-score baby				

Problems with hypermobility? _____ Yes / No

If so, how would it manifest? _____

_____

Before the pelvic problems, have you experienced:

A difference in leg lengths   Yes / No   Diagnosis/Symptoms: _____

_____

Knee complaints   Yes / No   Diagnosis/Symptoms: _____

_____

Foot complaints   Yes / No   Diagnosis/Symptoms: _____

_____

Hip complaints   Yes / No   Diagnosis/Symptoms: _____

_____

Lower back pain   Yes / No   Diagnosis/Symptoms: _____

_____

Neck complaints   Yes / No   Diagnosis/Symptoms: _____

_____

Have you been injured in an accident or a fall?   Yes / No

Diagnosis/Symptoms: _____

Have you participated in a lot of sports?   Yes / No

Which? _____

When? _____

Have you had physiotherapy before?   Yes / No

For what condition? _____

When? _____

Is a physiotherapist currently treating you?   Yes / No

For what condition? _____

Are you being treated by a chiropractor?   Yes / No

For what condition? _____

How many treatments have you had? _____

Is there ongoing therapy? _____

What method(s) is/are being used? _____

What have been the results? _____

Is a specialist treating you?   Yes / No

For what condition? _____

Examination

Posture
Inspection of the Patient in the Standing Position 1

Posture	Dorsal	Ventral	Lateral

Inspection of the Patient in the Standing Position 2

	Left	Right
Femoral condyles endorotated		
Leg length		
Feet position		
Weight bearing		

Remarks

❏ Palpation of the posterior superior iliac spine (PSIS) while the patient is standing is not a reliable test, but with experience you will be able to gain a sense of the position of the ilia. Meanwhile, make the patient bend forward and then return upright to help you gain even more of a sense of the position.

❏ If the femur is more in internal rotation and the PSIS on the same side is higher, this could suggest an inflare and anterior rotation of the ilium, which positions the hip joint more ventrally.

Inspection of the Patient in the Supine Position

Position of the hips	Asymmetric leg posture	Pelvic asymmetry	Deviation of the trunk

Remarks

Use neurological tests to rule out other causes of pelvic pain such as a damaged disc or sciatica.

Functional Passive Examination of Hip/SI Joints

Tests Performed with Patient in the Supine Position
Stability Test for the Pelvis

Active straight-leg raising (ASLR) may reveal a noticeable difference in pain between the left and right leg, which improves if a pelvic sling or compression is used at the level of the trochanter on both sides. Ask the patient which leg feels heavier. To make it possible to lift one leg, one needs to tilt the opposite ilium forward (on this side a "counternutation" of the sacrum takes place) and tilt the ilium on the side that is lifted backward (here a "nutation" of the sacrum takes place). This means that the sacrum makes a 3D-rotational motion.

Hip Tests

	Left			Right		
	Range	Pain score	Endfeel	Range	Pain score	Endfeel
External rotation						
Internal rotation						
Abduction						
Adduction (from abduction to the starting position)						
Flexion						
Extension (from flexion to the starting position)						

SI Tests

	Left	Right
Resistance against hips in adduction (gapping SI joints)		
Passive external rotation hip with 90° flexed hip and knee		
Passive internal rotation hip with 90° flexed hip and knee		
Iliolumbar ligament (hip in maximal abduction, 90° flexed with bent knee, apply pressure on the knee in the direction of the buttocks)		
Sacrotuberal ligament (hip in maximal flex with bent knee, knee in the direction of the ipsilateral shoulder, apply pressure in the direction of the buttocks)		
Sacrospinal ligament (hip in maximal flex with bent knee, knee in the direction of the contralateral shoulder, apply pressure in the direction of the buttocks)		
Patrick's Sign (place the left foot on the right knee and bring the left knee to the floor or bed surface; this tests the left SI joint); fix the right ilium		

Tests Performed with Patient in the Side-Lying Position

Testing the Coordination in Stabilizing the Pelvis (Static-Resisted Testing)

Do not score strength but rather pain or ability to stabilize the pelvis.

	Left	Right
Resistance against hip extension = backward-tilting ilium		
Resistance against flexed hip = forward-tilting ilium		
Resistance against abducted hip = compression SI joints		
Resistance against extended knee = forward-tilting ilium		
Resistance against flexed knee = backward-tilting ilium		

Remarks

Backward-tilting ilium = nutation sacrum

Forward-tilting ilium = counternutation sacrum

Physiotherapy Diagnosis

Pain localized: _____

_____

_____

Observed dysfunction: _____

_____

_____

Functional limitations: _____

_____

_____

Social and other activities avoided: _____

_____

_____

Mental/emotional status: _____

_____

_____

Ability to perform activities of daily living (ADLs): _____

_____

_____

15

Therapy

Many experts consider use of a pelvic sling during pregnancy to be a suitable therapy for the treatment of PRP even though slings decrease the pain in only half the women who use them (Mens et al. 1996; De Groot and Van der Schoot 1996). The purpose of the sling is to prevent symptoms of pelvic instability from becoming worse, following the line of thought that patients seldom completely recover from the symptoms during pregnancy (Engelen et al. 1995; Mens et al. 1996).

However, a range of treatment options exists. The therapy methods I have described in this book have helped almost all of the pregnant women treated; 98 percent of the 430 women we followed experienced a benefit. Their pain was noticeably reduced and they became functional without use of a sling, crutches, or a wheelchair. Of the many hundreds of patients I have worked with, only a few did not respond to treatment. The sole aid that I use on a regular basis is an abdominal support or girdle during pregnancy, which helps to slightly lift the position of the baby.

The prognosis associated with the use of these exercises is very favorable. Within a few months patients can function normally, return to work or sports, and work out. A small percentage of patients have needed to come back after delivery for additional treatment. Research has found that with a conventional approach, 35 percent are symptom free within a month after birth, but 7 to 18 percent have serious complaints up to eighteen months after delivery (Ostgaard et al. 1991). Less than 2 percent (n = 7) of the women we treated during pregnancy still had serious complaints eighteen months after delivery. Of those seven women, five were at the end stage of a next pregnancy or had recently delivered. The sixth woman experienced postnatal depression, and the seventh had stopped the treatment and home exercises after two sessions and had never again undertaken any other treatment or self-treatment.

Many of the patients whom I treated while they were pregnant have since become pregnant again. Most of them came in for therapy, as we had agreed, in the early part of their subsequent pregnancy. At the very first symptom, they came in for a refresher on the exercises needed to restore pelvic symmetry. All these pregnancies proceeded nicely; the symptoms were kept well under control. The women worked out and resumed participation in sports activities.

In general, my treatment proceeds on the following hypotheses:

❑ Complaints are not the result of instability, but rather are caused by a misalignment of the pelvis. A three-dimensional twisting of the pelvis causes pain and dysfunction.

❑ Therapy must first concern itself with correcting the position of the ilia; only after this correction can the entire pelvic area be stabilized.

❑ The best way to help the patient is by teaching her repositioning techniques that can be performed at home, either alone or with the help of her partner.

❑ During and after pregnancy the stabilizing function of the abdominal muscles is somewhat compromised (Gilleard et al. 1996). As a result, the sacrum may slide forward in the pelvic ring due to the forward movement of the trunk in relation to the legs (Don Tigny 1995). Other stabilizing muscles or more stable postures can be used to keep the sacrum in its normal place.

❑ By using correct posture, in which the weight rests on the heels, the nutated sacrum is pressed against the ilia.

❑ Stabilizing the pelvis requires compressing the SI joints, either manually or with muscular force or both, during activity and during rest.

❑ Principles of form and force closure can be used to improve stabilization. Pelvic stabilization should take place on an ongoing basis, day and night; this is made possible by assuming certain postures and using the right muscles.

Treatment

General Guidelines

Calm the patient. A patient with pelvic pain has probably been overwhelmed by the intense pain and frustrated by the challenge of trying to perform her daily activities. She is afraid to move and afraid for the future.

Explaining the situation can help alleviate some of her fear and fixation on the idea that the pain is going to be permanent. Using a model of the pelvis, let her see what the problem is and why it's important that her pelvis be symmetrical. Explain why she will have to exercise frequently, and confirm with her that she will realistically be able to undertake an exercise regimen.

Tell the patient that the way to keep the pelvis from twisting and to prevent pain is to strengthen the stabilizing hip muscles (the extensor and external rotator muscles) and to relax the inner thigh muscles (adductor muscles).

Encourage your patient to continue to exercise after the in-office therapy sessions end. This is very important for the continued success of the therapy. The last pain often disappears when the patient's condition allows her to work out. Don't treat the patient too often; once a week is sufficient. This also allows her time to exercise on her own. Ultimately, the patient must do most of the work herself.

Trust in the therapy begins the moment the patient understands what's involved and instinctively feels the logic of what you're saying.

Symmetry and Stabilization Exercises

The goal of the exercises is to restore function to the pelvis, hips, and spine. The lessening of pain is the natural result of restoration of function.

The *symmetry exercise* (Figure 5.2 on page 31) is meant to halt the twisting of the pelvis and can be used as therapy during or after pregnancy. It takes time for the exercise to work; an experienced therapist can feel when things are returning to normal.

When assisting with the symmetry exercise, the best results are obtained by using a continuous, light, oscillating movement applied with little pressure (see Figure 5.2C). The direction in which the force is supplied is very important; follow the arrows depicted in Figure 5.2C. Certain postures or movements may be painful, particularly moving from a position with knees outstretched as far back as possible to a closed-leg position. When the ilia move back to the closed-leg position, they tend to move laterally away from the sacrum if the stabilizing muscles are not yet in control. Repetitions of these exercises must be guided until the therapist is sure the patient can move her legs from her hips without pain or with much less pain. When the pain subsides it means coordination of the stabilizing muscle system is returning. Do not end the treatment sessions until such movement is no longer painful. You can use muscle energy techniques or other mobilization techniques to hasten this process.

Note the following pointers:

❑ The direction of pressure is in an oblique line aimed at the floor (dorsal, cranial, lateral).

❑ If there is still pain after the hip movement is no longer blocked, change the direction of pressure to cranial and slightly more medial.

Remember that this mobilization is meant to reposition the ilia at the SI joints; it is not meant as a gapping of the pubic symphysis or as an overmobilization of the hip joints. Therefore, do not just move dorsally, which would endanger the hip joint, but *always* use a cranial component. If you follow the given directions you will notice that when total hip movement is relaxed (some women can stretch quite extensively yet still feel that something is blocked), the endfeel of the movement changes, and you will be able to sense the endfeel of the SI joint.

At the moment the legs can spread their full width and can move back and forth without pain, you have realigned the ilia and sacrum, and independent hip movements are possible again. Independently of the intensity or duration of the ilium subluxation, this can be achieved in one or more treatments. Sometimes it happens with one click, within a few minutes. Sometimes it takes as many as five treatments of approximately a half hour each.

When the pelvis is out of balance, the facet joints and discs of the lower back may have dysfunction as well. To relax the lumbosacral area, the physiotherapist moves the pulled-up knees in a quick rhythm from left to right, using a small supple movement, after which the legs are spread again.

If the patient continues to experience pain even though she has accomplished spreading and closing the hips, a blockage may still exist. This could mean that one ilium is not tilted in the right way. Try the following exercises from Chapter 6: "Exercise for a Painful Leg" (see page 46), "Exercising with Assistance" (see page 46), and "Relieving a 'Locked' Pelvis" (see page 47). This last exercise is identical to tests of the sacrotuberal and sacrospinal ligaments. The stretching of the ligaments strongly stimulates the proprioceptive sensors. When the SI joint recovers, nutation is again possible.

It is only after pelvic and hip symmetry are restored that the patient is prepared to follow the coordinated exercise program.

The *stabilization exercise* (see Figure 5.3 on page 34) can be attempted as soon as the patient does not find it painful or uncomfortable to perform, often after the first treatment. If it takes longer, do not worry. Just be patient.

While doing the stabilization exercise, which is performed standing, make sure the knees are slightly bent and the feet are placed apart. Re-establishing balance—until the muscle tension in the back diminishes—should start at the ankles. The pain should diminish if the patient is distributing her weight properly. In the correct position, the ilia are tilted toward the posterior and the sacrum is slightly arched forward. To improve the coordination of the stabilizing muscle system, make the patient stop in the middle: right-middle-left-middle, etc. The stabilization exercise must be done frequently, whenever the patient is standing.

After these two exercises, it can be very useful to stabilize the pelvis, preferably with the help of the muscles that cause external rotation or abduction: the hip abductors and the buttocks. Stabilization of the lower back is also needed. According to research from the University of Queensland (Hodges and Richardson 1997, 1998, 1999), the lumbar spine relies for stability on the muscles that actively support the area. Four mechanisms are used for support: tension from the thoracolumbar fascia, intra-abdominal pressure, the paraspinal muscles, and the deep lumbar extensors (multifidi). The lumbar multifidi, the paraspinal muscles, and the internal oblique and transverse abdominal muscles are needed to stabilize the lower back. The timing of activation of this muscular system is especially important. Cocontraction of the transverse abdominal and multifidi muscles has to occur prior to any movement of the limbs. Stabilization of the total lumbopelvic area relies as well on compression of the SI joints by force or form closure, as described earlier. If you take a closer look at all the illustrations in this book, you will notice that either the participation of the stabilizing muscles or the principle of form closure is required in every posture and exercise.

Patients do not need a pelvic sling for support if they use their muscles in this preventive manner. The patient's anxiety diminishes when she knows how to reduce the pain. Anxiety is also reduced when she is once more able to use her joints and when coordination returns.

Compression of the SI Joints

The moment the planes of the SI joints are restored to their proper position, the application of compression on the joint becomes very important. This is achieved through either mechanical forces (e.g., legs apart in sitting; carefully chosen side-lying postures in which the ilium compresses the sacrum) or muscular forces. Without compression, the ilium will again shift out of alignment. Compression is needed to hold the ilia in place and also acts in a prophylactic manner. Once the position of the ilia has been stabilized, joint use improves and muscles are reactivated. As a result, the joints are brought back to their normal function in the body.

SI Joint Compression Through Posture Exercises

Standing

Standing stabilization exercises (see Chapter 5) promote a rhythmic compression of the SI joints. The result is better mobility in the joints, restored leg and pelvic-floor control, and an increase in the tension of the hip abductors and hip external rotators. By flexing the knees slightly, the hamstring muscles are engaged, positively affecting the angle and compression of the pelvis. Hamstring engagement produces a loading of the sacrotuberal ligament and a posterior pelvic tilt, which results in sacral nutation, in which the sacral base nods forward. This is the most stable position for the pelvis; in it, the sacrum is less likely to slip from the pelvic circle. During this exercise, body weight should be borne primarily by the heels; the toes are free to move.

Sitting

The sitting position also offers an opportunity to compress the SI joints. Sitting in the tailor's position or with legs crossed noticeably lessens the tension in the oblique stomach muscles (see Chapter 8; Snijders et al. 1995).

If while sitting one pays close attention to this compression by abducting the hips, it is possible to get the spinal column to move independently of the pelvis. This can compensate for a dysfunctional pelvis or weak, overstretched abdominal muscles, and the spinal column can move normally.

Lying Down

Other positions that promote secure contact between the sacrum and ilium include lying on one's side with a cushion between the legs and lying on one's back with knees and legs turned outward.

SI Joint Compression Through Muscle Activity

Back and leg muscles can be used to strengthen SI joint compression. The self-bracing SI joint compression model offers excellent approaches for therapy. The muscles this model focuses on are labeled in Figure 15.1. If the muscles defined in the model as stabilizing are first trained in coordination and later in strength, the restoration of pelvic function will be well on its way.

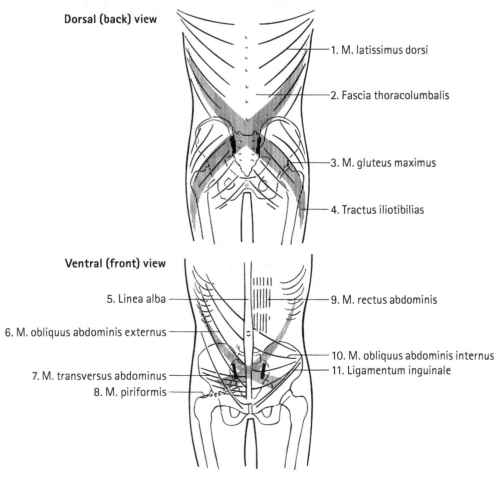

Dorsal (back) view

1. M. latissimus dorsi
2. Fascia thoracolumbalis
3. M. gluteus maximus
4. Tractus iliotibilias

Ventral (front) view

5. Linea alba
6. M. obliquus abdominis externus
7. M. transversus abdominus
8. M. piriformis
9. M. rectus abdominis
10. M. obliquus abdominis internus
11. Ligamentum inguinale

15.1. Muscular stabilization of the pelvis and lower back
(SOURCE: Snijders, Nordin, and Frankel 1995)

In this illustration you can see that the biomechanics of the pelvis involve both the back and leg muscles. Muscles on the plane of the SI joints are burdened when these bones shift out of proper position. Tensing of the fascia thoracolumbalis plays an important role in stabilization of the pelvis and lower back. Muscles that are attached to the fascia therefore play an important role in forming the stabilizing system patients can use. This system of transverse and oblique muscles that crosses the SI joints plays a part in the compression of the SI joints, which help to counteract any shifting.

What can be done if the transverse or oblique abdominal muscles cannot be used for stabilization? This may occur during pregnancy when the angle at which the abdominal muscles pull on the pelvis becomes less favorable (Gilleard et al. 1996; Mens 1996). It can also occur when these muscles are still weak after delivery.

In this situation it can be painful to use the adductor muscles to stabilize the pelvis. Attempts to contract the adductors can pull at the already swollen pubic symphysis, resulting in misalignment if only one adductor is pulling. Nutation and force closure in the horizontal plane offer one solution. The ilia must tilt backwards to make the sacrum nutate. The gluteus maximus and the biceps femoris, via the sacrotubal ligament, can help achieve this (Vleeming et al. 1995, Don Tigny 1995). Try to prevent inhibition of the gluteus maximus by preparing the pelvic area first: Use abduction and external rotation in the basic posture if the trunk wants to tilt forward. Then, the pull of gravity will take effect and movement diminishes through a self-bracing mechanism that is set in motion by nutation. Nutation provides tension on the dorsal interossal ligaments and the sacrotuberal ligaments, through which more friction-compression and a bigger capacity (the ability to hold one's body upright against the pull of gravity) come into existence for the pull of gravity (Vleeming et al. 1990).

Every irritation or dysfunction of the SI joints can inhibit the gluteus maximus. Weak buttock muscles can affect how one walks and can overtax the hamstrings. If this continues, the result may be instability in the SI joint (Lee 1996). Consequently, it is important to keep the buttock muscles strong to prevent chronic pelvic instability. Align the pelvis again if there is pain, so that such irritation can be prevented.

There is an association between PRP and sports that involve frequent hip adduction and internal rotation. A movement in which the legs are forcefully closed stretches the dorsal ligaments of the SI joints. It is possible that this is how the potential inflare mobility is advanced and outflare dysfunction is originated.

The pelvis should be brought into balance so that the external rotators and abductor muscles can perform their stabilizing function. Also, it is important that the buttock muscles be used as much as possible when the patient turns in bed, stands up, walks at a normal pace, and climbs stairs. Compression of the SI joints via the dorsal structure occurs when one tenses the fascia thoracolumbalis via the gluteus maximus, the latissimus dorsi, and the erector spinae.

While walking, the pelvic girdle is laterally stabilized through the gluteus medius and minimus and the contralateral adductor muscles. As one leg is lifted, the hip abductors function in harmony with the gluteus maximus; this action should stabilize the pelvis on the horizontal plane (Don Tigny 1995). In the case of instability, these muscles are inhibited by overuse of the pelvic-floor and inner thigh muscles. The patient tries to compensate by displacing the body's center of gravity above that joint—compensated as in the Trendelenburg test to lessen the shifting forces in the joint (Lee 1996). This braking disappears as the ilium is repositioned with symmetry exercises and the muscles are trained with stabilizing exercises. One major advantage of the stabilization exercises is that the stance is transformed into an active form—the patient is continuously compressing the SI joints, just as in walking. The knees are lightly bent to involve the biceps femoris and to activate the nutation of the sacrum.

While a person is sitting, form closure on a horizontal plane entails external rotation of the hips; this may or may not be in combination with abduction (Snijders et al. 1995). Form closure of the pelvis is essential during pregnancy because in a seated position the adductors and oblique abdominal muscles should perform the force closure (Vleeming et al. 1995). As discussed earlier, this is not always possible during pregnancy (see Figure 13.2B on page 101).

Exercising during pregnancy has many advantages. It lessens anxiety, returns self-confidence, and prepares the woman for delivery. And last but not least, exercising makes the mother-to-be realize that she has to be healthy and strong to take care of her family. Health is very precious and much more important than anything else.

16

After Pregnancy

Delivery

Delivery plays an interesting role in the recovery of pelvic pain. Pain diminishes immediately after delivery in a large group of women, but in some women pain increases following delivery. Other women do not experience any pain during pregnancy but begin having pain during or immediately after delivery. We investigated many factors related to delivery in our published studies, but found only two factors (amount of pain and duration of delivery) to be of significant importance in their effects on PRP.

During delivery the sacrum tilts forward (nutation) to allow the distance between the pubic bone and coccyx to expand as much as possible. In a difficult delivery nutation needs to be maximized. To make this happen, sometimes the woman pulls her legs up toward her torso. A danger exists if the woman pushes her legs against the hands of two helpers who try to keep the legs bent. If this occurs, the pelvic canal will become somewhat smaller rather than larger, impeding delivery. Further, she may be applying differing amounts of force with her two legs. In addition, if two people are holding her legs and applying different amounts of pressure, it may create the risk of pelvic wringing.

To correct these various problems, symmetry and stabilization exercises (Chapter 5) can be done immediately after delivery. I did this myself following my own delivery and have directed many of my patients to do so, and so have others who experienced intense pelvic pain in the first few days after delivery. The result is an instant lessening of the pain. Then, the patient can lie down, stand, and walk with little or no pain. As a result, pain medication is often no longer necessary. Do not be afraid that the pubic symphysis will be ruptured by the abducted posture called for in the symmetry exercise. The spreading of the legs is not felt in the area of the pubic symphysis, but in the lower back or sacro-iliac area.

The second or third treatment does not have to be given in patients' homes, because patients are usually in good enough shape by then to travel to the physiotherapist's office for treatment. This has been the case with the patients I have treated. After one or two months they also began to take part in fitness-related activities.

Whenever possible, it is important to restore symmetry before the delivery. Of the approximately 430 patients we followed who did this exercise program during pregnancy, about 75 percent had a natural delivery without the help of vacuum extraction, forceps, Caesarean section, or induction. If the pain worsens after delivery, we advise patients to contact us as soon as possible so we can proceed with the therapy described earlier. A small percentage of women came back for treatment a few times in the first months after delivery. Within six months postpartum, almost all the women we treated were functioning normally again, although 10 percent still experienced some pain or dysfunction a year later. Of the 430 women we followed, 18 percent had experienced another pregnancy or delivery.

We have had to treat only a few women for longer than three months. Now we know that these women benefit the most from a six-week multidisciplinary approach combining manual therapy, sports, and psychological care for emotional disturbance, work-related problems, and family background.

Fitness Advice

When a patient is able to do all the exercises in this book, it's time for her to begin a regular fitness program. The tips provided here are based on the premise that the physiotherapist will be able to guide the patient with the help of exercise equipment found in a gym or other exercise space.

Women who still have complaints need to be individually coached. Depending on the severity of the complaints, the following regimen will take place either in a few weekly sessions or over a period of months. When a numbered step can be completed without triggering extra pain in the days following the exercise session, you can move on to the next numbered step. Through trial and error, determine what combination best suits your patient.

1. Begin training the latissimus dorsi, the buttock muscles, and the oblique/transverse abdominal muscles without any extra weight.

2. Next, move to music. Include side steps and other warming-up dance moves for as long as the patient feels like it.

3. Then add stretching exercises.

4. Now you can add heavier conditioning training or aerobics and abdominal exercises.

5. Finish with more stretching exercises and relaxation techniques.

What to Pay Attention To

General

❑ Let patients take part in group exercise whenever they desire and for as long as their comfort level allows.

❑ During exercise, guide your patients to focus on how it feels. Teach women to listen to their bodies so they know how much they can do. Forget about counting to a certain number or exercising for a certain time span, even if not much is accomplished. Let the patient lead.

❑ Make sure the pelvis is properly aligned before training begins so that women can sit securely with the ilia tilted slightly backward.

❑ Learn to limber up the pelvic floor. There are many ways to teach this, for instance by using breathing techniques. Relaxing the pelvic floor is more important than strengthening it. Coordinating movements is key in recovery; strength comes later.

❑ Never train the hip adductors when women still have complaints of pelvic pain!

❑ When stretching, ensure that the thigh doesn't turn inward; this will cause the ilium to move away from the sacrum and the pain to return.

❑ If the patient experiences pain in her pelvis during the exercises, she should lie down on an exercise mat and do her symmetry exercises until the pain diminishes enough for her to continue working out.

Once this program can be fully completed without pain, the patient can move on to using exercise equipment. How long it takes to reach this point will differ from patient to patient.

Weight Training

- ❑ When using weight machines, begin by using the least amount of weight possible (or no weight at all, if desired).

- ❑ On some types of equipment, the handles are attached to the middle of a foot pedal. To use this sort of device, one needs to have very flexible hips. Avoid this type of equipment at first.

- ❑ Instruct the patient never to clamp her legs together or around an object.

- ❑ Advise patients to sit on exercise equipment with their ankles crossed.

- ❑ When getting on or off equipment, watch the position of the legs; keep them spread widely.

- ❑ After working out, encourage patients to take a long, hot shower or visit the sauna to reduce the likelihood of sore muscles or pain.

- ❑ Residual pain is possible, but only at acceptable levels. If there is more than minimal pain, patients should cut back on their training.

In the beginning, working out once a week is desirable; in this way, a woman learns what her limits are and what kind of pain to expect. For the long term, two or three workout sessions a week is even better.

Prognosis

Most patients may experience pelvic pain again around the time of menstruation (72 percent) and during a subsequent pregnancy (85 percent; Mens et al. 1996).

If the complaints take place during menstruation, I recommend that the patient use medication to control the pain so that she can continue to move normally, rather than letting cramps immobilize her and risking the remembering or reexperiencing of pelvic pain.

During a subsequent pregnancy, carefully follow the stabilization exercises prescribed during the preceding pregnancy. The joints become stiffer with age, so the problems of instability disappear over the course of a woman's life. The prognosis is quite positive if patients remember the basic principles involved: Realign the ilia whenever pain returns, and establish an exercise regimen as soon as the symptoms disappear.

References

Albert, H., M. Godskesen, and J. Westergaard. 2001. Prognosis in four syndromes of pregnancy-related pain. *Acta Obstet Gynecol Scand* 80:505–10.

Albert, H., M. Godskesen, J.G. Westergaard, T. Chard, and L. Gunn. 1997. Circulating levels of relaxin are normal in pregnant women with pelvic pain. *Eur J Obstet Gynecol Reprod Biol* 74(1): 19–22.

Bjorklund, K., T. Naessen, M. Nordstrom, et al. 1999. Pregnancy-related back and pelvic pain and changes in bone density. *Acta Obstet Gynecol Scand* 78(8): 681–5.

Bjorklund, K., M.L. Nordstrom, and S. Bergstrom. 1999. Sonographic assessment of symphyseal joint distention during pregnancy and postpartum with special reference to pelvic pain. *Acta Obstet Gynecol Scand* 78(2): 125–30.

Bjorklund, K., M.L. Nordstrom, and V. Odlind. 2000. Combined oral contraceptives do not increase the risk of back and pelvic pain during pregnancy or after delivery. *Acta Obstet Gynecol Scand* 79(11): 979–83.

Brynhildsen, J., A. Hansson, A. Persson, and M. Hammar. 1998. Follow-up of patients with low-back pain during pregnancy. *Obstet Gynecol* 91(2): 182–6.

Buyruk, H.M., H.J. Stam, C.J. Snijders, J.S. Lameris, et al. 1999. Measurement of sacroiliac joint stiffness in peripartum pelvic pain patients with Doppler imaging of vibrations (DIV). *Eur J Obstet Gynecol Reprod Biol* 83(2): 159–63.

Centraal Bureau Statistieken, "Enquete Beroeps Bevolking" [Official Dutch Statistics from the Profession Questionnaire of 1997].

Damen, L., H.M. Buyruk, F. Guler-Uysal, et al. 2002. The prognostic value of asymmetric laxity of the sacroiliac joints in pregnancy-related pelvic pain. *Spine* 27(24): 2820–4.

De Groot, V., and J.T.M. van der Schoot. 1996. Bekkeninstabiliteit in de zwanger-schap [Pelvic instability in pregnancy]. *Profundum* 3:21–3.

Don Tigny, R.L. Mechanics and treatment of the sacroiliac joint. 1995. In *The integrated function of the lumbar spine and sacroiliac joints,* A. Vleeming, V. Mooney, T. Dorman, et al. (eds.). Symposium November 9–11, 1995, San Diego, Rotterdam; 515–29.

Engelen, M.J.A., et al. 1995. Bekkenpijn en zwangerschap [Pelvic pain and preg-nancy]. *Ned Tijdschr Geneeskde* 139:1961–4.

Gilleard, W.L., et al. 1996. Structure and function of the abdominal muscles in primigravid subjects during pregnancy and the immediate postbirth period. *Phys Ther* 76:750–62.

Greenman, P.E. 1995. Clinical aspects of sacroiliac function in walking. *Low back pain and its relation to the sacroiliac joint.* In proceedings from The Second Interdisciplinary Congress on Low Back Pain in Relation to the Sacro-Iliac Joint in San Diego, California. 353–9.

Hansen, A., D. Vendelbo Jensen, M. Wormslev, et al. 1999. Symptom-giving pel-vic girdle relaxation in pregnancy. *Acta Obstet Gynaecol Scand* 78:111–5.

Hansen A., D. Jensen, E. Larsen, et al. 2005. Postpartum pelvic pain—The 'pel-vic joint syndrome': A follow-up study with special reference to diagnostic methods. *Acta Obstet Gynecol Scand* 84:170–176.

Hodges, P.W., and C.A. Richardson. 1998. Delayed postural contraction of trans-versus abdominis in low back pain associated with movement of the lower limb. *J Spinal Disord* 11(1): 46–56.

Hodges, P.W., and C.A. Richardson. 1997. Relationship between limb movement speed and associated contraction of the trunk muscles. *Ergonomics* 40(11): 1220–30.

Hodges, P.W., and C.A. Richardson. 1999. Transversus abdominis and the su-perficial abdominal muscles are controlled independently in a postural task. *Neurosci Lett* 265(2): 91–4.

Johnston, R.C., and G.L. Smidt. 1969. Measurement of hip-joint motion dur-ing walking: Evaluation of an electrogonimetric method. *J Bone Joint Surg* 51A: 1083.

Johnston, R.C., and G.L. Smidt. 1970. Hip motion measurements for selected activities of daily living. *Clin Orthop* 72:205.

Kihlstrand, M., B. Stenman, S. Nilsson, et al. 1999. Water gymnastics reduced the intensity of back/low-back pain in pregnant women. *Acta Obstet Gynecol Scand* 78(3): 180–5.

Kristiansson, P., K. Svardsudd, and B. von Schoultz. 1996. Back pain during pregnancy: A prospective study. *Spine* 21(6): 702–9.

Larsen, E.C., C. Wilken-Jensen, A. Hansen, et al. 1999. Symptom-giving pelvic girdle relaxation in pregnancy I: Prevalence and risk factors. *Acta Obstet Gynaecol Scand* 78:105–10.

Lee, D. 1996. Instability of the sacro-iliac joint and the consequences to gait. *The Journal of Manual and Manipulative Therapy* 1:22–9.

Lee, D.G. 1999. *The Pelvic Girdle*. Edinburgh, Scotland: Churchill Livingstone.

MacLennan, A.H. 1991. The role of the hormone relaxin in human reproduction and pelvic girdle relaxation. *Scand J Rheumatol Suppl* 88:7–15.

MacLennan, A.H., and S.C. MacLennan. 1997. Symptom-giving pelvic girdle relaxation of pregnancy, postnatal pelvic joint syndrome and developmental dysplasia of the hip. *Acta Obstet Gynecol Scand* 76(8): 760–4.

Mens, J.M., A. Vleeming, C.J. Snijders, et al. 2001. Reliability and validity of the active straight-leg raise test in posterior pelvic pain since pregnancy. *Spine* 26(10): 1167–71.

Mens, J.M., A. Vleeming, C.J. Snijders, et al. 2002. Responsiveness of outcome measurements in rehabilitation of patients with posterior pelvic pain since pregnancy. *Spine* 27(10): 1110–5.

Mens, J.M., A. Vleeming, C.J. Snijders, et al. 1999. The active straight-leg raising test and mobility of the pelvic joints. *Eur Spine J* 8(6): 468–74.

Mens, J.M., A. Vleeming, C.J. Snijders, et al. 2002. Validity of the active straight-leg raise test for measuring disease severity in patients with posterior pelvic pain after pregnancy. *Spine* 27(2): 196–200.

Mens, J.M.A. 1994. Bekkeninstabiliteit in en na de zwangerschap [Pelvic instability in and after pregnancy]. Een tussentijds rapport. *Cesar* 25:4–5.

Mens, J.M.A. 1995. Bekkenpijn door zwangerschap; een nieuwe aandoening? [Pregnancy related pelvic pain; a new disorder?] *Ned Tijdschr Geneeskd* 139: 1964–6.

Mens, J.M.A. 1996. Bekkeninstabiliteit [Pelvic instability]. *Kwartaaluitgave nvom* 4:153–60.

Mens, J.M.A., et al. 1996. Understanding peripartum pelvic pain. *Spine* 11: 1363–70.

Noren, L., S. Östgaard, G. Johansson, et al. 2002. Lumbar back and posterior pelvic pain during pregnancy: a three-year follow-up. *Eur Spine J* 11(3): 267–71.

Östgaard, H.C., and G.B.J. Andersson. 1992. Postpartum low-back pain. *Spine* 17:53–5.

Östgaard, H.C., et al. 1991. Prevalence of back pain in pregnancy. *Spine* 16: 549–52.

Östgaard, H.C., et al. 1993. Influence of some biomechanical factors on low-back pain in pregnancy. *Spine* 18:61–5.

Östgaard, H.C., G. Zetherström, and E. Roos-Hansson. 1997. Back pain in relation to pregnancy: a six-year follow-up. *Spine* 22(24): 2945–50.

Pool-Goudzwaard, A.L., M.C. Slieker ten Hove, M.E. Vierhout, et al. 2005. Relations between pregnancy-related low back pain, pelvic floor activity and pelvic floor dysfunction. *Int Urogynecol J Pelvic Floor Dysfunct* 16(6): 468–74.

Röst, C.C., J. Jacqueline, A. Kaiser, A.P. Verhagen, and B.W. Koes. 2004. Pelvic pain during pregnancy: A descriptive study of signs and symptoms of 870 patients in primary care. *Spine* 29(22): 2567–72.

Röst, C.C., J. Jacqueline, A. Kaiser, A.P. Verhagen, and B.W. Koes. 2006. Prognosis of women with pelvic pain during pregnancy: A long-term follow-up study. *Acta Obstet Gynaecol Scand* 85:771–77.

Röst et al. Risk factors of pregnancy-related pelvic pain. (Working paper to be published).

Skaggs, C.D., H. Prather, G. Gross, J.W. George, P.A. Thompson, and D.M. Nelson. 2007. Back and pelvic pain in an underserved United States pregnant population: A preliminary descriptive survey. *Manipulative Physiol Ther* 30(2): 130–4.

Schoellner C., N. Szöke, and K. Siegburg. 2001. Pregnancy-associated symphysis damage from the orthopedic viewpoint: Studies of changes of the pubic symphysis in pregnancy, labor and post partum. *Z Orthop Ihre Grenzgeb* 139(5): 458–62.

Schwartz, Z., et al. 1985. Management of puerperal separation of the symphysis pubis. *Int J Gynaecol Obstet* 23:125–8.

Snijders, C.J., et al. 1993. Transfer of lumbosacral load to iliac bones and legs, part I: Biomechanics of self-bracing of the sacro-iliac joints and its significance for treatment and exercise. *Clin Biomech* 8:285–94.

Snijders, C.J., M. Nordin, and V.H. Frankel. 1995. *Biomechanica van het spierskeletstelsel.* Utrecht, The Netherlands: Lemma.

To, W.W.K., and M.W.N. Wong. 2003. Factors associated with back pain symptoms in pregnancy and the persistence of pain two years after pregnancy. *Acta Obstet Gynaecol Scand* 82:1086–91.

Turgut, F., M. Turgut, and M. Cetinsahin. 1998. A prospective study of persistent back pain after pregnancy. *Eur J Obstet Gynecol Reprod Biol* 80(1): 45–8.

Van Gelder, R. 1997. Vrouwen zitten er mooi mee [Women and their sitting habits]. *Fysioscoop* 23(2): 22–4.

Van Vugt, A.B. 1998. Is bekkeninstabiliteit oplosbaar? [Is pelvic instability solvable?] *Profundum* 1:14–7.

Vleeming, A., et al. 1990. Relation between form and function in the sacroiliac joint, part 2: Biomechanical aspects. *Spine* 15:133–6.

Vleeming, A., V. Mooney, C. Snijders, and T. Dorman. 1992. *First interdisciplinary world congress on Low back pain and its relation to the sacroiliac joint.* Rotterdam: Eco.

Vleeming, A., V. Mooney, T. Dorman, et al. (eds). 1995. *The integrated function of the lumbar spine and sacroiliac joints.* Symposium November 9–11, San Diego, Rotterdam.

Vleeming, A., et al. 1995. A new light on low back pain. In *The integrated function of the lumbar spine and sacroiliac joints,* A. Vleeming, V. Mooney, T. Dorman, et al. (eds.). Symposium November 9–11, San Diego, Rotterdam; 149–68.

Wang, S.M. 2003. Backaches related to pregnancy: The risk factors, etiologies, treatments and controversial issues. *Curr Opin Anaesthesiol* 16(3): 269–73.

Wu, W., O.G. Meijer, C.J. Lamoth, K. Uegaki, J.H. van Dieen, P.I. Wuisman, J.I. de Vries, and P.J. Beek. 2004. Gait coordination in pregnancy: Transverse pelvic and thoracic rotations and their relative phase. *Clin Biomech* 19(5): 480–8.

Wu, W.H., O.G. Meijer, K. Ugegaki, et al. 2004. Pregnancy-related pelvic girdle pain (PPP), I: Terminology, clinical presentation and prevalence. *Eur Spine J* 13(7): 575–89.

Resources

When researching this topic on the Internet, suitable terms to use in search engines include lumbopelvic stabilization, sacroiliac, SIJD, pubic symphysis, pelvic instability, pelvic girdle pain, tailbone, coccygodenia, subluxation, pregnancy, hypermobility, chronic pain syndrome, core stability, and pelvic floor dysfunction.

Websites

On the Internet there are many sites that describe the symptoms of pregnancy-related pelvic pain but that present clinical guidelines that differ partly or completely from those described in this book. Be aware that many of the theories and pieces of advice you can find on the Internet are not evidence based.

Reliable medical research can be found on the following websites:

www.pubmed.gov

www.medline.cos.com

www.medscape.com

For additional information, including a list of certified physical therapists and a DVD for health-care practitioners demonstrating the therapy techniques, visit the author's website at **www.rosttherapy.com.**

How to Test Yourself

The following text is repeated from Chapter 2 for easy reference. Are your symptoms caused by pelvic instability? A patient with pregnancy-related pelvic pain due to misalignment of the pelvis may have problems with the following exercises:

Test Exercise 1

- ❏ Lie down on your back and stretch out your legs.
- ❏ Try to lift one leg and then lower it.
- ❏ Then try lifting the other leg.

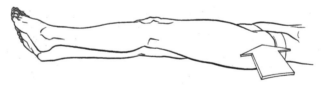

1. Does pushing inward against your hips make it easier to lift one leg?

If this exercise is difficult, if it hurts, or if you can't even lift your leg in this position, try to lift your leg while pressing against your hips with your hands. Use your hands to exert pressure on both sides of your hips, as if you were pushing your hips together.

If you notice that it is easier to lift your leg when you press your hands into your hips, your symptoms are probably caused by pelvic instability. If applying pressure to both sides of your hips does *not* help you to lift your leg, it may be a good idea to consult your doctor.

Test Exercise 2

Standing, try to move a light object, such as a piece of paper, forward along the floor with your foot. When pelvic instability or injury is present, this exercise will often be easier with one leg than the other.

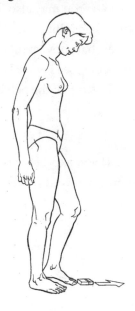

2. Difficult!

Test Exercise 3

- ❑ Lie on your back with your legs outstretched.
- ❑ Bend your knees but keep your feet flat on the floor.

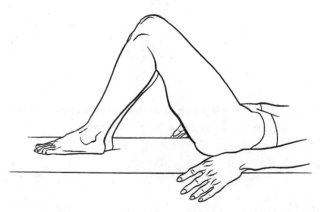

3. Is it difficult to spread your bent legs while lying on your back?

☐ Try to move your knees apart while keeping the sides or soles of your feet together.

For someone with pelvic pain, this exercise can range from uncomfortable to extremely painful. You may experience the pain in the pubic bone or on the inside of the thighs near the groin. You may also feel pain in the lower back on either side, at one of your sacroiliac joints (due to joint compression or resistance to normal sacroiliac or lumbar movement). If you frequently experience pain in the tailbone area (the coccyx, see Figure 1.1 on page 8), this exercise may cause you to feel tension in the bottom of the pelvis.

Test Exercise 4

Sit on a hard chair for a while. If you experience pain in your tailbone, it could be caused by tension in the bottom of your pelvis. Most pelvic pain patients can only sit for a limited period of time.

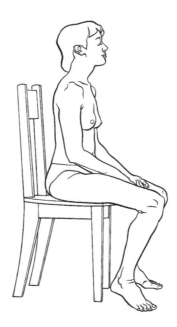

**4. Sitting on a hard chair without experiencing pain
is usually only possible for a short period of time.**

Index

A

abdominal muscle exercises, 38–39

abdominal muscles, separation of, 36

abdominal support during pregnancy, 118

Acta Obstetricia et Gynecologica Scandinavica, 89

active straight-leg raising (ASLR) test, 103, 110, 114

activities of daily living, difficulties with, 12–13

activities of daily living, recommendations for: bicycling, 64, 66, 74; changing your baby, 70–71; climbing stairs, 64; doing laundry, 66; driving, 64, 65; getting dressed, 62–63; holding a baby on your lap, 72; making love, 69–70; picking up a baby, 71; picking up your child from bed, 70; shopping, 68; standing up, 62; sweeping, 66, 67, 75; swimming, 66, 68; turning over in bed, 68–69; turning to one side, 63; using a baby carrier, 72–73; using a stroller, 73; using child car seats, 74–75; vacuuming, 66, 67, 75

adductor muscles, tension in, 9, 20, 75, 125

anti-phase pelvis-thorax coordination, 108

anxiety, 22, 23

at-home exercises: abdominal muscles, 38–39; back muscles, 37–38; buttock muscles, 42; circulation and pelvic-floor muscles, 43–44; for coordina-

tion, 42–43; exercycling in a standing position, 45; forward stretch, 41; for locked pelvis, 47; for painful leg, 46; side muscle stretch, 44–45; spinal stretch, 40–41; spinal twist, 40

B

baby carrier, use of, 72–73

back muscle exercise, 37–38

back muscles, anatomy of, 124–125

back pain: chronic, 4, 9, 99; gestational, 6, 89

ball cushion, 58

bicycling, 13, 45, 64, 66, 74, 75

bladder function, 58

bloating, 13

breathing for childbirth, 79

Buttinger, Christine, 22, 23–25

buttock muscles, 125, 126

buttock muscles stretch, 42

C

Caesarean section, 24, 79, 128

case history, sample, 110–114

changing table, recommended, 75

child car seats, use of, 74–75

child care: bicycling with your baby, 74; changing your baby, 70–71, 75; holding a baby on your lap, 72; picking up a baby, 71; picking up your child from bed, 70; tips for, 76; using a baby carrier, 72–73; using a stroller, 73, 75; using child car seats, 74–75

childbirth: assisted labor, 16, 20; and

Printed in the USA
CPSIA information can be obtained
at www.ICGtesting.com
JSHW052018140824
68134JS00027B/2535